Brain Health Action Plan

Brain Health Action Plan

*Simple, Science-Backed Lifestyle
Changes that Optimize Cognitive Fitness
and Reduce Alzheimer's Risk*

TERYN CLARKE M.D.

Brain Health Action Plan © Copyright 2024 Teryn Clarke

All rights reserved. No part of this publication may be reproduced, distributed, or transmitted in any form or by any means, including photocopying, recording, or other electronic or mechanical methods, without the prior written permission of the publisher, except in the case of brief quotations embodied in critical reviews and certain other noncommercial uses permitted by copyright law.

The resources in this book are provided for informational purposes only and should not be used to replace the specialized training and professional judgment of a health care or mental health care professional.

Neither the author nor the publisher can be held responsible for the use of the information provided within this book. Please always consult a trained professional before making any decision regarding treatment of yourself or others.

The advice and strategies found within may not be suitable for every situation. This work is sold with the understanding that neither the author nor the publisher is held responsible for the results accrued from the advice in this book.

ISBN: 979-8-89316-309-4 (Hardcover)
ISBN: 979-8-89316-310-0 (Paperback)
ISBN: 979-8-89316-311-7 (Ebook)
ISBN: 979-8-89316-323-0 - (Audiobook)

Before You Start

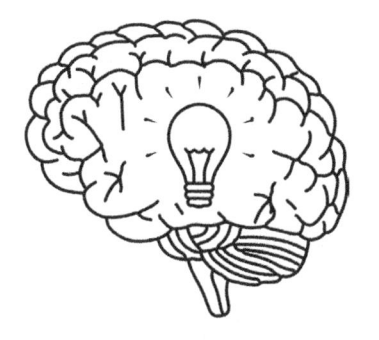

Go to
www.brainhealthactionplan.com/checklist
to download a copy of the tasks and habits
in this book to check off as you go!

This book is dedicated to . . .

My husband: you are generous of spirit beyond measure. I am so lucky to get to spend my life with you.

My kids: your patience, kindness, and support mean the world to me.

Liz and Sue: two amazing women who were able to look past the ugly realities of Alzheimer's disease and continued to visit their dear friend until her last days.

My mom: I wish we knew all of this fifty years ago.

CONTENTS

Foreword xi
Chapter 1: Get Ready to Improve Your Brain Health 1
Chapter 2: Betty's Story 8
Chapter 3: Understanding Alzheimer's Disease 12
Chapter 4: Goals, Tasks, and Habits 23
Chapter 5: Terry's Story 34
Chapter 6: Nourishing Your Brain 41
Chapter 7: Sugar, Sweet Saboteur 61
Chapter 8: The Toxicity of Seed Oils 89
Chapter 9: Time-Restricted Eating 100
Chapter 10: Prepare for Success 111
Chapter 11: Optimal Sleep 116
Chapter 12: Get Moving 139
Chapter 13: Education and Exercising Your Brain 152
Chapter 14: How General Health Affects Brain Health ...161
Chapter 15: The Mind-Brain Connection:
　　　　　　Stress, Spiritual Wellness, and Depression 190
Chapter 16: Avoiding Toxins 203
Chapter 17: Recipes 212
Appendix A: Protein 229
Appendix B: Fiber 231
Appendix C: Streak Tracker 233
Acknowledgements 235

FOREWARD

By Dr. Joseph Ladapo
Author of *Transcend Fear: A Blueprint for
Mindful Leadership in Public Health*
Professor, University of Florida College of Medicine
Surgeon General of Florida

I met Dr. Teryn Clarke in the summer of 2020 during the peak of the COVID-19 pandemic's lockdowns, school closures, mask zealotry, and fear. Brought together by a mutual friend, Dr. Simone Gold, we participated in an America's Frontline Doctors' event in Washington, D.C. and joined several other physicians who believed the pandemic was being severely mismanaged. The doctors provided livestreamed education about public health, the adverse health and social impacts of school closures, psychological and emotional tolls of lockdowns and fear-based decision making, and treatment strategies for COVID-19 that they were successfully using with their own patients. That gathering ended with a press conference in front of the U.S. Supreme Court, as members of the group—Dr. Clarke and I included—took turns sharing a few words with a small audience. There were probably no more than two dozen people in the crowd, but within just a few hours, that press conference would reach tens of millions of people worldwide. The explosive, grassroots dissemination of the video served as incontrovertible evidence that masses of people in the United States and abroad were hungry for truth and authenticity, and innately aware that their governments were not being honest with them. The other wonderful consequence of our gathering that day in Washington, D.C. was the opportunity to meet courageous, virtuous, and heart-centered people like Dr. Teryn Clarke.

In her most recent book, *Brain Health Action Plan*, Dr. Clarke draws on her deep and extensive experience as a board-certified neurologist and clinical researcher to help Americans better understand how to reduce their risk of developing Alzheimer's disease. The content she shares is as valuable as the delivery; her book will be accessible to virtually every American, and her suggestions about changes we can make to our diets, lifestyles, and environments are delivered in a way that is invaluable to and easily digestible by all.

Reading her book reminded me of an important lesson I've learned over my years of practicing medicine, which is that there are two distinct types of doctors:

On one end of the spectrum are the doctors who rigorously apply the scientific knowledge they've learned to patient care, with little deviation. These doctors can treat common conditions, but will be less successful when patients' complaints are nonspecific, or when diseases take an atypical or unexpected turn. That's because these doctors aren't blessed with the ability to integrate wisdom about health, wellness, and humanness into their scientific knowledge and expertise.

On the other end of the spectrum are doctors who are blessed with an intuition for healing, and naturally integrate the wisdom they've accumulated from life and from their clinical experience into patient care. These doctors have the ability to recognize when a "recommended" treatment may actually make the patient worse rather than better, or that a patient's complaints about fatigue or pain may require a more holistic treatment plan that considers his life circumstances, relationships, stress level, diet, or work rather than a simple test for thyroid function. Because their goal is comprehensive health rather than merely "treatment," physicians like this develop deep and powerful relationships with their patients, and are often able to communicate about health in a way that can help patients attain a degree of understanding that is both actionable and powerful. Dr. Clarke is this type of physician, and in this book, she shares with the reader her gift of powerful communication strategies for improving health and reducing dementia risk.

While I enjoyed every chapter of the book, I particularly appreciated her discussion about toxic substances in our environment, because it ties together so much of what we currently face in the battle for freedom for humanity and freedom from oppressive forces. It is ironic—but perhaps inevitable—that the comforts of life we enjoy in this modern age, which have contributed to our longevity, eased our suffering, and smoothed the physical challenges of human existence, have also brought with them an environment teeming with molecules that disrupt our DNA, interfere with our cellular biology, and upset our physiology. Nearly worldwide, humanity is forced to contend daily with toxins in our water, toxins in our air, toxins in our food, toxins in our clothing, and toxins in our homes. Many of these toxins accumulate in our bodies, and some of these toxins, such as per-and polyfluoroalkyl substances (PFAS), have been shown to be present in virtually every adult living in this country, based on National Health and Nutrition Examination Survey (NHANES) studies, and likely impair immune function and increase cardiovascular risk. Other toxins, such as organophosphate insecticides, are likely reducing sperm concentrations in men (with potential repercussions for reproduction of the species)—and heaven knows what else.

Our bodies are under constant assault from our modern environment, and my experience as a physician and clinical researcher has taught me that people have different degrees of ability to process these toxins and attenuate their harms, with some people far more sensitive than others.

We are seeing more action and attention to the presence of toxic exposures, such as with the FDA's recent crackdown on PFAS in food packaging, but federal and state policies that attempt to regulate and diminish these exposures are no match for how broadly they have permeated our lives. And while a healthy debate could be had about which toxic exposures may be worth their risks (for example, there is currently a debate about ethylene oxide, which is used to sterilize medical equipment), the real focus of our attention as human beings should be on the fact that many of these toxic exposures exist or persist because the underlying force—indeed, the frequency that defines the medical and pharmaceutical industries—is greed.

As humans, there is so much good that we embody, express, and share with others: our love, our selflessness, our courage, our ingenuity, our curiosity, our kindness, and our genius. But unfortunately, much of what shapes the structure of our lives and our world is fueled by forces with a much lower vibration: greed, insecurity, lust for power, and fear.

Sometimes these forces play out in the open. The overreaction of the U.S. government during the COVID-19 pandemic is one example. Those darker, lower vibrational forces inspired separation, isolation, fearfulness, opportunism for individuals seeking political power, and sweeping assaults on individual freedom and sovereignty. Sometimes these forces play out in the shadows. For example, when trans fats, which are produced from the industrial process of hydrogenation of vegetable oils, were first introduced in the early 1900s, manufacturers gravitated toward them because they extended shelf life of baked goods. Decades later, we learned that this convenience caused innumerable premature deaths from cardiovascular disease worldwide.

TERYN CLARKE M.D.

A major step toward reclaiming our lives and wresting our destinies out of the hands of corporations and governments—the ones whose first priorities are their own survival and growth rather than the survival and growth of human beings—is elevating our consciousness. One path for reaching that goal—and perhaps the only one accessible for nearly all humans—is shedding the stress and trauma that entwines our souls, interacts with our epigenetics, and hinders the oneness within us and our relationship with the universe.

Five years ago, I was unaware of this knowledge and had no conscious experience in this area. But around that time, thanks to my wife Brianna, I had the good fortune of working with Christopher Maher, a former Navy Seal with training in Chinese medicine theory, as well as other talents and gifts from God, and permanently healing myself from much of the stress and trauma that burdened my soul. This work freed me from the shackles that stress and trauma create and empowered my consciousness to rise and experience more and more of the oneness that, as our souls already know, is our shared destiny.

This type of freedom is far more powerful than the selfish interests that poison our environments and contribute to diseases like Alzheimer's, cancer, heart disease, chronic fatigue, and autoimmune disease, and helps us understand our own motivations, interests, and goals with more clarity. Free people can more easily recognize the influences of manipulation and more easily identify the forces at play in our lives that are completely invested in self-interest rather than the interest of humanity.

We are living through an exciting and profoundly interesting time in history, and I believe it will grow even more interesting as time passes and more light and understanding permeate human consciousness. I believe that eventually, we will learn to navigate and expand our formidable power as creator beings, and thus completely and permanently advance our interests over the interests of selfish governments and corporations.

Our health is an important part of this journey, and I wish you all good health and hope you enjoy and learn from Dr. Clarke's wonderful book.

CHAPTER 1

Get Ready to Improve Your Brain Health

Someone in the US is diagnosed with Alzheimer's disease every minute.[1] As a board-certified neurologist and someone who has had a family member impacted by this disease, I have seen Alzheimer's up close for two decades. I designed this book to help you do everything in your power to avoid this devastating disease.

There is no shortage of books explaining Alzheimer's disease. There is also no shortage of books with broad, sweeping advice on how to reduce your risk. You might be asking, *Is this just another book filled with medical jargon and vague suggestions for improving my health?*

My answer to you is no. Most books on the topic provide information with the hope that you will figure out how to make changes. *Brain Health Action Plan* is different. It will help you set small, attainable goals that will turn into lasting healthy habits.

Who Is This Book For?

You are in the right place if you are worried about memory loss and are ready to do something to prevent it. The book is perfect for you if you have a family member with Alzheimer's disease and you are determined to change your lifestyle and get your brain as far away from Alzheimer's disease as possible. It's also the book for you if you found out that you have a gene that increases your risk for Alzheimer's, and you want to learn how to beat your genetics.

Maybe you already know what you need to do to lower your risk for Alzheimer's disease but need help with the steps to get there. Let's face it: there is a lot of information out there on lifestyle choices that promote brain health. The challenge is how to go about changing your lifestyle. In this book, we'll go step by step, adding small habits that make a big difference in brain health.

Why I Wrote This Book

Ten years ago, I started emphasizing lifestyle optimization for my patients with **Alzheimer's disease and related dementias**. I have seen a handful of patients embrace dramatic lifestyle changes, reverse their memory problems, and graduate from my clinic. This is, unfortunately, very rare.

The problem is that brain deterioration starts decades before symptoms appear. That means that the time to address risk factors is by midlife. Because no meaningful treatment for dementia exists, you've got to prevent it from happening in the first place.

Brain health research has exploded in the past couple of decades. The tremendous amount of information about what is good for the brain and what is bad for the brain can be both empowering and overwhelming. How do you incorporate all of this information so you can achieve brain wellness?

You need an action plan.

I wrote this book to boil down all the information. As you read, you'll learn **why** you need to make healthy changes, **how** to make changes, and why **today** is the day to start.

What You'll Learn

To take control of your brain health, you need to understand how the brain works and how to keep it healthy. With that background in place, we'll set up goals that will turn into healthy habits.

In Chapter 3, we're going to dig into brain function, Alzheimer's disease, and the processes that transform a healthy brain into a diseased one.

Chapter 4 explains how to set specific goals that you'll use to optimize brain health. Most chapters end with a "Take Action" section where you will use these strategies to adopt new healthy habits step by step.

In Chapters 6 through 8, we'll dive into nutrition. Unlike many books that focus primarily on taking things away, we'll start by adding brain-healthy foods that might be missing from your diet. Then we'll tackle sugar and how to cut it down with less sacrifice than you might expect. And have you heard about seed oils? We'll cover why they are toxic and how to avoid them. We'll perform a couple of pantry and refrigerator audits, reading the labels on the foods already in your home so you have an idea of which brands you want to continue to purchase and which ones you want to replace with a healthier option. Take that process at your own pace—one that reflects your health choices and budget. If you've been wondering why fasting has been getting so much attention in the brain health space and how it might benefit you, you'll get the answer in Chapter 9.

We spend about a third of our lives sleeping. We'll spend Chapter 11 discussing why sleep is critically important for brain health and how you can get more and better-quality rest.

Chapter 12 focuses on the importance of physical exercise, and Chapter 13 focuses on cognitive exercise. Both are necessary components of achieving ultimate brain health.

Chapter 14 addresses the profound brain dysfunction caused by vitamin deficiencies, dehydration, and other general medical conditions.

Chapter 15 explains the brain health effects of stress and depression, along with some initial steps to address them.

Chapter 16 is all about toxins. It includes a frank discussion about alcohol and smoking, how they damage the brain, and why it is important to minimize or avoid both habits.

The book concludes with some of my favorite brain-healthy recipes.

How to Approach This Book

I want you to succeed in optimizing your brain health. So, I've outlined a multitude of ways to reduce your risk of dementia. However, you can't tackle them all at once, and you don't need to tackle them in the order they are listed. You may read through the entire book once and then decide which healthy habits you will work on adopting first. Or, you may decide to read the chapters in the order that makes the most sense to you. I recommend starting with the chapters that cover improvements you think will be the easiest to make or where you are already probably pretty close to being optimized. For example, if you already exercise frequently, you might start with Chapter 12 to see if there are any tweaks you need to make or if you are already doing everything you need to do. Conversely, if you absolutely detest exercise, do not start with that chapter!

Improving your brain health is about making progress, not seeking perfection. There may be areas that you cannot optimize completely. Don't let that discourage you from making changes you are able to incorporate and sustain. As you work through this book, you might even surprise yourself. You could be thinking, *I have a terrible sweet tooth. I will never be able to cut down on sugar, so I'm going to skip that chapter and start working on sleeping better. A lot of the sleep mini habits look like they'll be easy for me to adopt.* The magic of building these small lifestyle habits is that they're all interconnected. For example, sleeping better can rebalance the hormones that govern appetite, which reduces cravings for sweets and carbohydrates. When you revisit the sugar chapter after optimizing sleep, you might find that crowding out sweets isn't as difficult as you expected.

You might choose to make just one or two sustainable lifestyle changes the first time you read this book. Maybe you'll decide to end screen time two hours before you go to bed most nights and drink a full glass of water daily right after your morning coffee. That's a great start. Those are two habits that will promote health and consistency.

Revisit the book and incorporate new tiny habits when you feel ready. For example, you can add more healthy activities during your screen-free hours at night—maybe a ten-minute meditation or a relaxing nightly cup of decaffeinated green tea. In the morning, you could add a five-minute walk after you finish your coffee and water. As you read through the book, all these mini habits will make sense. And remember to be kind to yourself if you miss a day or stumble back to old habits. That's human.

Now that you know what's in store, let's improve your brain health.

Notes

[1] "Alzheimer's Disease Facts and Statistics," The Fisher Center for Alzheimer's Research Foundation, 2020, https://www.alzinfo.org/understand-Alzheimers/Alzheimers-disease-facts-and-statistics/.

CHAPTER 2

Betty's Story

"You need to fix my brain!" Betty announced as she walked into my office and handed me a pile of medical papers.

She was lean, not quite five feet tall, and clad in leopard-print yoga pants and trendy sneakers. She reminded me of the feisty and fit grandmas I've seen on Instagram doing kettlebell swings and box jumps. At eight-seven, she was starting to notice some mild memory changes, and she wanted no part of it.

She ran marathons earlier in life, and she still walked 5Ks. This lucky lady had never had much of a sweet tooth. I thumbed through the medical papers she had brought with her. Her medical history was simple—few medications, not many diagnoses. But when I got to her labs, I was stunned.

Betty had two copies of the ApoE4 gene, which accelerates the risk of developing Alzheimer's disease. People with her genetic pattern are ten times more likely to get Alzheimer's disease than the average person. In other words, nearly everyone with her genetic pattern shows signs of

Alzheimer's disease by the time they turn eighty. I would have expected her to have come to my office at least seven years sooner. Yet here she was, charging into my clinic at age eighty-seven with only minor memory problems. How had she beaten her genetics?

The Secret to Her Success

I've seen a handful of patients who, like Betty, were sharper than I expected for their age and genetics. Their stories were similar: they each exercised consistently and didn't overindulge on sweets. Without knowing it, they were living a brain-healthy lifestyle. These folks inspire me. They are convincing proof that the best way to stay sharp and stave off dementia is to focus on healthy living.

Betty is an inspiration, but don't let her choices intimidate you. You don't have to start running marathons or completely swear off your favorite sweet treat. I would encourage you, however, to assess your lifestyle and find areas where you can make small but meaningful improvements.

Understanding the Genetic Risk of Late-Onset Alzheimer's Disease[1]

Earlier in the chapter, I mentioned that Betty had two copies of the ApoE4 gene. With the invention of home genetic testing, people who do tests like 23andMe may be confronted with the knowledge that they have one or two copies of this gene but not know what it means or what to do about it.

The apolipoprotein E (ApoE) gene is the most common measurable genetic risk factor for late-onset (after age sixty-five) Alzheimer's disease. All of us have two copies of the ApoE gene: one from our mother and one from our father. The most common version, or allele, of this gene in the global population is the ApoE3 allele (usually abbreviated to E3), so the most common ApoE genetic profile is E3/E3. In this group, about 50% of individuals show signs of Alzheimer's disease by age eighty-five. The concerning gene is the E4 version. Having this gene seems to accelerate the progress of Alzheimer's disease so that people with one or two copies of the E4 allele will most likely have symptoms of Alzheimer's disease earlier. In individuals who have one copy of this accelerator allele and thus the genetic profile E3/E4, the 50% prevalence of Alzheimer's disease moves to age eighty. For individuals with an E4/E4 genetic profile, the prevalence of Alzheimer's symptoms is estimated to be between 75% and 95% by age eighty, which means almost everyone with this genetic profile has Alzheimer's disease by age eighty.

Your brain health at any given age is the sum total of your genetics plus everything your brain has been exposed to throughout your life. As we age, we have more cumulative exposure to poor diet, toxins, sedentary living, insufficient nutrients, and the list goes on.

There is a saying regarding Alzheimer's disease that "genetics load the gun, and environment pulls the trigger." A loaded gun poses a threat but doesn't cause damage unless someone pulls the trigger.

You may have a family history of Alzheimer's disease or E3/E4 or E4/E4 genetics that have "loaded the gun" to increase your risk of late-onset Alzheimer's disease. If this describes you, I'm right there with you. The prospect of getting Alzheimer's disease is terrifying. This information can feel defeating and overwhelming.

I choose to take my strong family history of Alzheimer's disease as a call to action, and I hope you will too. We have the power to make healthy lifestyle choices that lower our risk of triggering Alzheimer's disease. Adopting healthy habits in each of the major lifestyle areas—nutrition, exercise, education, sleep, stress and mood, and toxins—can keep our brains healthy much longer than our genetics or family history might suggest.

NOTES

[1] Early-onset Alzheimer's disease is diagnosed under age sixty-five. It is rare and runs in some families due to several specific gene mutations. Families in which this disease runs are usually aware of this disease and under the care of a neurologist and a geneticist. The bulk of research on Alzheimer's disease risk factor modification has focused on the much more common late-onset form, which is also the focus of this book.

CHAPTER 3

Understanding Alzheimer's Disease

How do our lifestyle choices influence our risk of Alzheimer's disease? To appreciate the connection, we need to understand what Alzheimer's disease is, the five brain-damaging core processes that cause it, and how lifestyle regulates those processes.

Alzheimer's Disease

Brain cells, called **neurons**, gradually die off throughout our lifetime. That's the natural process of aging. Alzheimer's disease occurs when the neurons are damaged and die off at a faster rate. This damage goes on in the background for decades before symptoms appear. At some point, the brain suffering from Alzheimer's disease doesn't have enough neurons to function normally, and that's when we start to see symptoms of dementia. The parts of the brain that usually dip below that critical threshold first are the short-term memory structures called the hippocampi. (That's the plural for *hippocampus;* there's one on each side of the brain.) This causes forgetfulness, which is often the first sign that someone may have Alzheimer's disease.

The term "Alzheimer's disease" was coined in 1910, three years after Dr. Alois Alzheimer published a paper describing a fifty-one-year-old woman who died from dementia. At autopsy, Dr. Alzheimer found an abnormal buildup of two proteins in her brain: beta-amyloid and tau. These proteins contribute significantly to the dysfunction and death of neurons. In the century since his discovery, scientists have determined that inflammation, oxidative stress, neurotransmitter imbalance, and vascular disease are additional core processes in the development of Alzheimer's disease.

Core Processes

Lifestyle choices connect to the risk of dementia by influencing the core processes that damage the brain. Let's explore each process in detail to better understand how they function. At the end of each explanation, we'll preview which lifestyle habits can influence these fundamental processes.

Toxic Proteins: The Plaques and Tangles of Alzheimer's Disease

Beta-amyloid and tau are two proteins that can form toxic clumps in the brain. Beta-amyloid clumps are called plaques, and they build up between cells in the brain. Because of their location, they can block communication between neurons and distort the structure of the brain. Beta-amyloid also triggers inflammation, which can kill nearby neurons.

Tau protein clumps are called tangles. Unlike beta-amyloid clumps, the tau clumps build up *inside* the neurons. They interfere with the normal cellular machinery inside the neurons and prevent them from functioning properly. As neurons start to fill up with tau clumps, they send out distress signals that trigger inflammation in the brain. The tangles continue to grow and eventually get so large that they cause the neuron to burst and die.

Lifestyle modifications aimed at reducing beta-amyloid include eating adequate protein, reducing sugar intake, getting adequate deep sleep, managing stress, treating high blood pressure, and practicing time-restricted eating. Lifestyle modifications aimed at reducing tau include getting adequate deep sleep and practicing time-restricted eating.

Inflammation

Inflammation is a key player in Alzheimer's disease. Brain injury, infection, and abnormal proteins like beta-amyloid and tau trigger the brain's immune system to fight. It releases inflammatory chemicals called cytokines to battle invaders. Once a bacterial or viral invader is defeated, the brain's immune system cleans up the debris from the battle, and the inflammatory reaction stops. It's a similar story with trauma – once the damaged brain tissue is removed by the immune system, inflammation ceases. The inflammatory story can end differently when the invader is beta-amyloid or tau. If these proteins are folded improperly (which we'll discuss in detail in Chapter 6), they may be resistant to breakdown, meaning that the brain's immune system can't defeat them. They persist indefinitely and continue to stimulate an immune reaction. In addition, the pace at which beta-amyloid and tau accumulate can overwhelm the brain's ability to clear the toxic proteins, meaning that the fight continues endlessly, causing chronic inflammation.

Widespread, chronic brain inflammation eventually damages the neurons, causing dysfunction and cell death. Chronic inflammation can also damage the blood-brain barrier (BBB), the protective layer that separates the brain from the bloodstream. When the BBB is impaired, toxins and immune cells from other parts of the body can enter the brain, causing further brain damage and perpetuating the cycle of chronic brain inflammation.

Lifestyle modifications aimed at reducing inflammation include drinking green tea, reducing sugar intake, reducing seed oil intake, practicing time-restricted eating, exercising, reducing stress, sleeping better, reducing alcohol intake, and quitting smoking.

Oxidation: Brain Rust

We're familiar with rust. It's what happens when metal is oxidized. But did you know that brain cells can also be oxidized? Doctors and scientists don't call this process brain rust. They call it oxidation or oxidative stress. Isn't it fitting that we describe ourselves as feeling rusty when we aren't functioning at our best?

The oxidative stress story starts with cellular metabolism—how cells make energy. Cells have tiny power plants inside them called **mitochondria** (that's plural for mitochondrion, an individual human cell can contain hundreds to thousands of mitochondria). The mitochondria take in nutrients and oxygen, then turn them into energy and free radicals. These free radicals are a natural byproduct of energy production, but they can be harmful because they carry an electrical charge.

When you were a kid, did you ever charge yourself up with static electricity by rubbing your socks on the carpet so you could give a shock to the first person you touched? That's a similar concept, except the shock that free radicals give off can cause permanent damage to any part of the cell they bump into—DNA, proteins, and even the mitochondria themselves. Free radicals can also kick off chain reactions that amplify their damaging power by creating more and more free radicals.

Thankfully, our cells have a strategy for dealing with free radicals: **antioxidants**. Antioxidants soak up the destructive free-radical shocks without injury. They act like rodeo clowns in the cells. Similar to the way rodeo clowns distract raging bulls so they won't hurt a fallen bull rider, antioxidants distract free radicals so they won't hurt healthy parts of the cell. They run around the cell saying, "Look over here," to free radicals, distracting them from damaging the important parts of the cells and absorbing their shocks. When your antioxidants are abundant, you have great cell protection from free radicals. The drawing below represents part of a cell that has adequate antioxidants to neutralize free radicals.

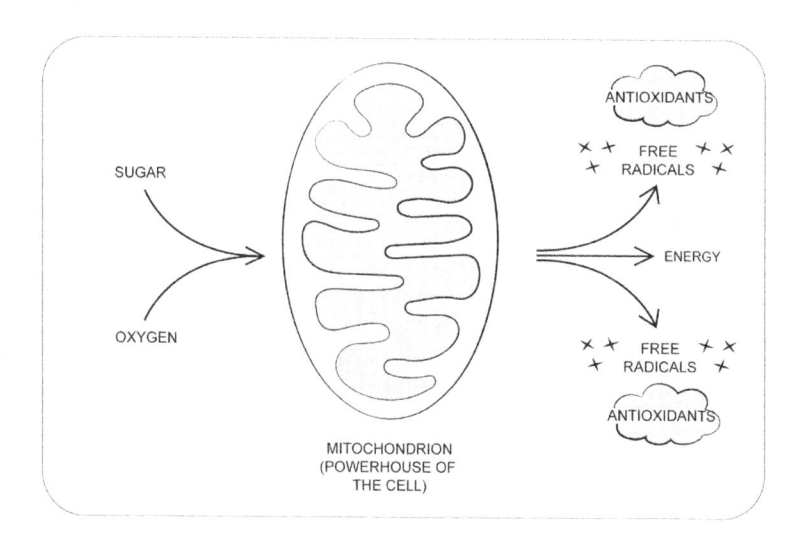

Oxidative stress happens when harmful free radicals outnumber helpful antioxidants. This can happen in any cell in the body, but the brain is more likely to get out of balance than other organs for two reasons. First, neurons naturally have lower antioxidant defenses than most other cells. Second, the brain is the most metabolically active organ in the body. It makes more energy than any other organ. High energy production means high production of free radicals. The diagram below shows part of a cell that does not have enough antioxidants to neutralize free radicals, putting it at risk of oxidation.

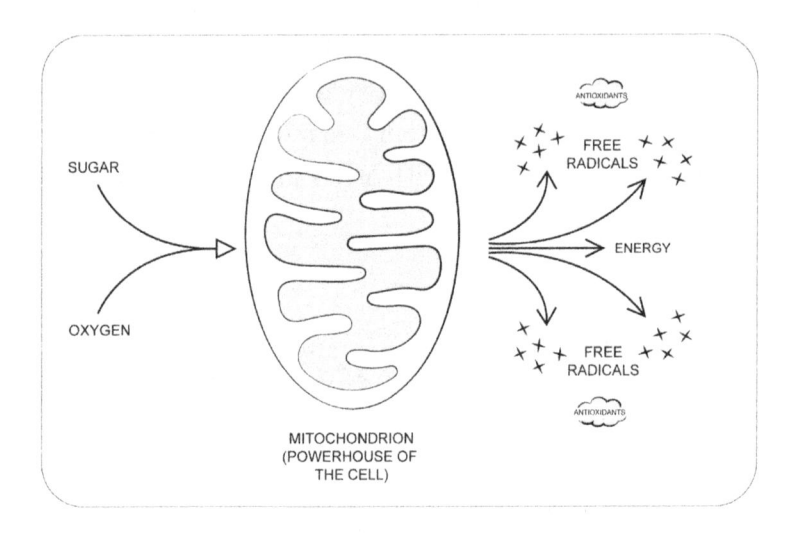

```
SUGAR ──┐
        ├──▶ [MITOCHONDRION] ──▶ FREE RADICALS (ANTIOXIDANTS)
OXYGEN ─┘                    ──▶ ENERGY
                             ──▶ FREE RADICALS (ANTIOXIDANTS)

MITOCHONDRION
(POWERHOUSE OF THE CELL)
```

Lifestyle modifications that target oxidative stress include drinking green tea; eating adequate protein, fruits, and vegetables; reducing sugar intake; reducing seed oil intake; reducing stress; sleeping better; reducing alcohol intake; and quitting smoking.

Neurotransmitter Imbalance

Neurotransmitters are chemicals that transmit signals between nerve cells in the brain and are crucial for proper brain function. When a neuron wants to communicate with another neuron, it releases neurotransmitters into the tiny gap between the neurons called the synapse. These neurotransmitters then travel across the synapse and bind to receptors on the neighboring neuron, sending signals that can either excite or inhibit the activity of that neuron.

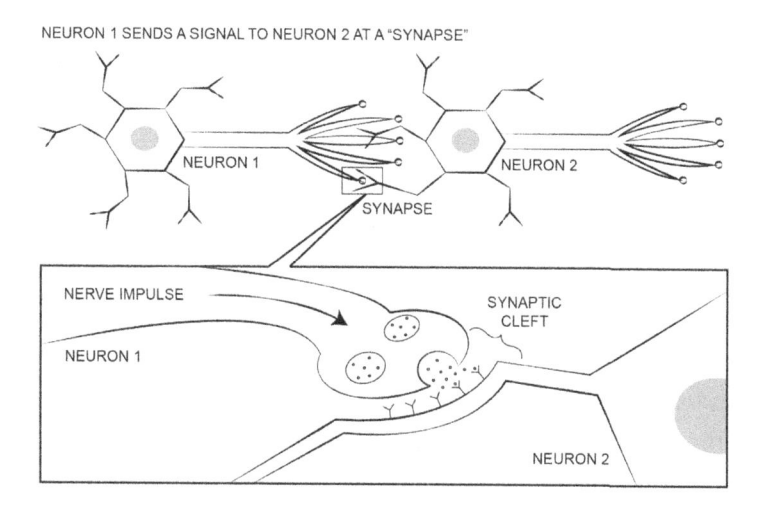

NEURON 1 SENDS A SIGNAL TO NEURON 2 AT A "SYNAPSE"

NEURON 1

NEURON 2

SYNAPSE

NERVE IMPULSE

NEURON 1

SYNAPTIC CLEFT

NEURON 2

The neurotransmitters we'll be discussing further are glutamate, gamma-aminobutyric acid (GABA), serotonin, dopamine, norepinephrine, and acetylcholine. When they are out of balance, communication between neurons is impaired, and you can suffer from symptoms such as fatigue, memory loss, and depression, to name a few. Clinical studies have identified that neurotransmitter imbalance is present in the brains of people who died with dementia.[1] For example, acetylcholine serves many functions throughout the nervous system. In the brain, it's involved in memory and learning. When it's low, we have trouble with both of those tasks. In fact, the brains of individuals with Alzheimer's disease show a significant decrease in acetylcholine, which results in cognitive decline. That's why the first medications to treat Alzheimer's disease were designed to increase acetylcholine.

Other neurotransmitters, like dopamine and serotonin, are important for mood regulation. Changes in these neurotransmitter levels lead to behavioral and psychological symptoms commonly seen in dementia, such as mood swings, depression, and agitation.

Lifestyle and health interventions aimed at restoring a healthy neurotransmitter balance include drinking green tea; eating adequate protein, fruits, and vegetables (including enough B vitamins and vitamin C); staying hydrated; reducing sugar intake; reducing seed oil intake; practicing time-restricted eating; exercising; reducing stress; sleeping better; reviewing medications with your medical provider; evaluating hormone levels; and reducing alcohol use.

Vascular Disease

The vascular system refers to the network of blood vessels that circulate blood throughout the body. Arteries deliver oxygen and nutrients to your organs. Veins carry away blood containing cellular debris and toxins. A healthy vascular system supplies optimal blood flow to the brain, allowing it to function well.

When the arteries supplying blood to the brain harden and fail, that is called cerebrovascular disease (*cerebro* = brain, *vascular* = blood vessels). Inadequate blood flow starves the mitochondria of the oxygen and nutrients they need to make energy for the neuron. This leads to an energy crisis in the neuron. The neuron starts to shut down, and it stops communicating with other neurons in the brain. Without adequate blood flow to carry away debris, toxins start to build up inside the neuron. If adequate blood flow is not restored quickly, the neuron dies.

Lifestyle and health modifications aimed at reducing vascular disease include working with your provider to assess and manage vascular risk factors like high blood pressure and high cholesterol, reducing sugar intake, and staying hydrated.

Lifestyle Influences the Core Processes

That was the bad news: toxic proteins, inflammation, oxidative stress, neurotransmitter imbalance, and vascular disease are the complex core processes that can damage your brain and lead to Alzheimer's disease. Here's the good news: you can make choices every day that lessen these processes.

Did you know that 40% of dementia is due to twelve modifiable risk factors? Scientists from around the world reported in 2020 that obesity, physical inactivity, low education, hypertension, smoking, depression, diabetes, hearing loss, infrequent social contact, air pollution, head injury, and excessive alcohol consumption are significant risk factors for Alzheimer's disease and related dementias.[2]

In their report, they encourage us to "be ambitious about prevention" because reducing these twelve risk factors through our day-to-day health and lifestyle choices might prevent or delay up to 40% of dementia.

We'll take a holistic approach to managing these risk factors by adopting mini habits in the following health and lifestyle categories: **nutrition, exercise, education, sleep, stress and mood, general medical health,** and **exposure to toxins.**

Notes

[1] Stuart G. Snowden, Amera A. Ebshiana, Abdul Hye, et al., "Neurotransmitter Imbalance in the Brain and Alzheimer's Disease Pathology," J Alzheimers Dis. 72, no. 1 (2019):35–43, https://doi.org/10.3233/jad-190577.

[2] Gill Livingston, Jonathan Huntley, et al., "Dementia prevention, intervention, and care: 2020 report of the Lancet Commission," Lancet 396, no. 10248 (August 2020):413–446, https://doi.org/10.1016/s0140-6736(20)30367-6.

CHAPTER 4

Goals, Tasks, and Habits

"The chains of habit are too weak to be felt until they are too strong to be broken."
—Samuel Johnson

In each of the following chapters, you'll create goals, accomplish tasks, and adopt habits that lead to improved brain health. Setting SMARTT goals (yes, there are two *T*s), streak tracking, habit stacking, crowding out, interrupting, and defining a self-reward system are tools that have propelled my patients toward success.

Goals and habits work hand in hand to help you grow and improve. When you set a goal, you're essentially laying out a road map for where you want to go. Habits are the vehicles that get you there. Every new healthy habit you adopt becomes a stepping-stone in building a routine that suits your goals and lifestyle. Setting goals and then aligning your habits with your health goals creates a powerful synergy that will propel you toward success.

SMARTT Goals

SMARTT (traditionally SMART) stands for Specific, Measurable, Achievable, Relevant, and Time-Bound. I've added the second T for Tiny. Creating SMARTT goals helps you focus, track progress, and stay motivated while working toward your brain health objectives. Let's take a closer look at each element:

- o **Specific**: Being precise about what you want gives your new habit a clear direction. Instead of just saying, "I want to exercise more," you'd say, "I will walk for twenty minutes every morning."

- o **Measurable**: Putting numbers into your goal helps you track your progress. Let's say your goal is to drink more water. You might set a measurable goal of drinking eight glasses of water a day.

- o **Achievable**: Keep it real, friend! Your goals should challenge you a bit, but they've got to be doable with the resources and abilities you have. If your goal is to read more, start by setting a realistic goal of reading for ten minutes a day rather than reading a novel a week.

- o **Relevant**: Make sure your goals matter to you. They should fit into the big picture of what you want to achieve overall.

BRAIN HEALTH ACTION PLAN

- **Time-Bound:** This can be either setting a deadline or setting a streak length. Tasks, like scheduling a visit with your doctor, may be more amenable to a deadline. For example, you could say, "I will call to schedule my yearly physical in the next week." Or, it can refer to how long you want to continue your new habit: "I'm going to walk for ten minutes every day for the next two weeks." The latter is also called a streak goal (see below) and can help you build positive habits.

- **Tiny:** By miniaturizing your goals, you're essentially making them less overwhelming and more achievable. Conquering small goals gives you quick wins that build momentum. Each little success boosts your confidence and motivates you to keep going. For example, if you don't exercise at all and your goal is to walk twenty minutes daily, consider breaking that down into bite-size chunks. So maybe start with five minutes a day. If you have a task to do, like a pantry audit to look for foods that contain seed oils (more on that in Chapter 8), set the goal to go through one category per week—salad dressings, cooking oils, or crackers, for example—instead of trying to remove all foods that contain seed oils from your entire pantry in one go.

Streak Goals

Streak goals are like a game in which your goal is to not break the chain of doing a particular thing. Think of it as your personal winning streak. They're about keeping a streak alive by doing something consistently, day after day. I recommend charting your streaks on paper or using a streak-tracking app on your phone. Checking off the task daily gives positive feedback, perpetuates your incentive, and makes the streak visual.

Let's say your streak goal is to meditate for ten minutes every day. The goal is to keep that meditation chain unbroken. Day one? You meditate. That's a mini goal achieved. Day two? Yes! You're working on a streak! And the days keep going, and you build an epic streak.

The longer your streak, the more you want to keep it going. Every day, you're beating your own record. Soon enough, that habit becomes so ingrained that you just naturally do it, like brushing your teeth or grabbing your morning coffee.

It's important to not beat yourself up if you miss a day. Life happens! The trick is to get right back on track. Streak habits are all about building consistency and creating habits that will last. If you find that you've dropped a habit for a while, setting a short streak goal can be a great way to start again. For example, if you've fallen out of the habit of exercise lately, set a short streak with a tiny goal: "I'm going to do one push-up daily for the next three days." Completing the streak provides a sense of accomplishment that stokes the fire of motivation.

Habit Stacking

Habit stacking is a great way to schedule healthy habits. We perform dozens of well-formed habits daily. One of the easiest ways to build a new habit is to tie it to one that you already have down pat. By linking a new habit to an existing one, you create a mental association that helps reinforce the new behavior. Think of habits you do automatically, like brushing your teeth, drinking coffee, checking email, or walking the dog. Trying to drink more water? Set a goal to drink a glass of water right after finishing your first cup of coffee. Increasing exercise? Take an additional lap of your morning dog walk or do five jumping jacks before you check your email.

The key is to keep it simple and realistic. When you pair small, manageable habits, they're more likely to stick than when you try to make a massive change all at once. Over time, as each habit becomes second nature, you can add more on top, creating a chain of healthy habits.

The Power of Crowding Out

Crowding out is a strategy you can use to build a lifestyle full of healthy habits. It involves adding something positive that will naturally push out something negative. It's a more forgiving and enjoyable way to make changes than focusing on giving up things. Instead of feeling like you're losing something, you're gaining new, healthier habits that promote a positive mindset. As you incorporate new, healthier habits, you start feeling better about your choices.

That makes it easier to phase out the old habits that no longer fit. Crowding out also tends to be more sustainable over the long term. Because you're integrating new habits gradually and are focused on the positive, your goals are less likely to be derailed by feelings of being overwhelmed or deprived.

In our day-to-day lives, we are often overfed yet undernourished. We'll take advantage of that mismatch to use brain-healthy foods to crowd out non-nutritious foods. When your body gets the fuel it needs, you'll have fewer cravings for unhealthy foods.

Here's an example of how crowding out works. Let's say you want to reduce your sugar intake. Instead of setting a goal of not having ice cream for four nights in a row, set a goal to have a bowl of fresh fruit for dessert four nights in a row. Instead of focusing on what you can't have, you turn the spotlight on adding healthy food that is delicious and satisfies your sweet tooth.

Healthy Interruptions

Interrupting is a helpful strategy for avoiding or delaying indulgences. It involves taking an intentional pause and adding a healthy step before indulging in an unhealthy temptation.

Here's an example: As I'm writing, the thought has popped into my head that I have toffee in the kitchen, and now

I'm craving it. I'm going to interrupt that temptation with a healthy choice. I'm craving toffee, but I'm going to have a bowl of berries before I eat the toffee. There are three possible outcomes in this scenario. The first one (which is what happened in this example) is that I had a bowl of berries and a glass of water. My sweet tooth was satisfied. After that, the toffee just didn't seem as appealing. The interruption ended up crowding out the sweet altogether. The second potential outcome could have been having the fruit and going on to have less of the toffee than I would have, had I gone straight to it without a healthy interruption. Think of that as a partial crowd-out. The last possibility would have been to have the fruit and then go on to have as much toffee as I would have had without an interruption.

Most of the time, the healthy interruption strategy leads to partially or completely crowding out the indulgence. On the rare occasions when we do go on to enjoy whole indulgence despite the healthy interruption, we still have added the healthy choice or behavior—such as an extra serving of fruit. Fortunately, the third outcome is the least common and least desirable of the three. Even so, it may still be a better result than not interrupting at all. All three scenarios result in adding a serving of fruit with all of its beneficial vitamins and antioxidants. However, healthy interruptions don't work for everyone. If you find that you consistently end up with option three, you may be adding too many calories to your day. In that case, skip this strategy and know that this book is loaded with plenty of other strategies to help you achieve optimal brain health.

Redesign Your Reward System

As you move through the chapters of this book, you're going to be setting and accomplishing a lot of goals and establishing many new habits. That is cause for celebration! It's worth taking a few minutes to think about how you reward yourself and check in on your relationship with food.

It's common to reward ourselves with food, which can create a tricky relationship with eating. If food is your go-to reward, it might influence your eating habits in a way that's not aligned with your new health goals. You might find yourself consuming unhealthy foods just for the sake of the reward.

There are many other ways to reward yourself that don't involve food. Celebrating achievements with activities or experiences can be just as fulfilling. If you have an unpleasant task to do, like working on taxes or cleaning the garage, determine your reward before you start it. You might decide that your reward will be watching an episode of your favorite streaming series, listening to music for fifteen minutes, reading a magazine, sitting outside for a bit, working on a hobby, or browsing the Web for an item you've been wanting. Anything not related to food will do!

Tasks

Some health goals are more amenable to tasks than habits, and some habits rely on a foundational task. When possible, breaking tasks into smaller chunks can be helpful. For example, if you're tackling the task of reviewing the side effects of the prescription and over-the-counter medicines you take (Chapter 12), consider breaking that into two separate tasks: review your prescription medications one week and your over-the-counter items the next week. Or break it up even further and review one medication a day until you've reviewed them all.

You're welcome to further miniaturize tasks if that works better for you. Just like habits, the smaller we make a task, the less likely we are to put it off, and our micro tasks will quickly lead to accomplishing goals.

Start with a Success Mindset

As you embrace new habits, set lifestyle goals, and start accomplishing your goals, your brain health will flourish. Envision what it will look and feel like when you have made meaningful changes. As you embark on this journey, adopt a mantra that helps you start your day on the right foot. Something like "I live a brain-healthy lifestyle." Or "I make brain-healthy choices daily."

Write it on a sticky note and put it on your bathroom mirror. Say it to yourself as you brush your teeth. The first moments are the rudder of the day: set your course for a day of brain-healthy choices.

Take Action: Tasks, Goals, and Mini Habits

Get ready to track your streaks

- ☐ Look at streak-tracking apps and the streak trackers in this book, then decide what you will use to help you build your new habits. Additional streak-tracking templates are available at www.brainhealthactionplan/streaks

Prepare for habit stacking

- ☐ Think about your day and write down all the things you do on a daily basis. Later, you can use this list to habit stack.

Redesign your reward system

- ☐ Spend 5 minutes thinking about when you reward yourself with unhealthy foods. Take a few more minutes and write down the foods you often use for a reward.
- ☐ Brainstorm a list of activities you enjoy. Seeing them on paper is the first step toward redefining your self-reward system.
- ☐ Commit to rewarding yourself with activities rather than food for one week, then two, and continue to build your streak until the habit is well-established.

Start with a success mindset

☐ Decide what your brain health mantra will be and write it on a sticky note.

☐ Put your sticky note in a place where you will encounter it first thing in the morning.

CHAPTER 5

Terry's Story

Terry was a firecracker.

She grew up in Hollywood in the 1950s, the product of North Dakotan parents whose early marriage was shaped by separation during World War II. She went to Hollywood High School with Linda Evans and Stephanie Powers. Terry was stunning: large hazel eyes, auburn hair, and the coveted hourglass figure of the era. Yet somehow, she maintained a girl-next-door approachability.

Terry was a kindergarten teacher and had a zest for life. Her friends described her as passionate about teaching kindergarten, skiing, and having a good time.

Terry raised her family in the 1970s and devoted more than full-time hours to her kindergarteners. This worked because the 1970s were the era of convenience foods. Fast-food and TV dinners allowed numerous commitments to coexist in a twenty-four-hour day. TV dinners got an upgrade to fancy freezer meals like Lean Cuisine, which fed American families without time wasted on cooking.

Terry always wanted to lose twenty pounds but never much more than that.

She drove a zippy red coupe that matched her personality. She loved that car, and somewhere in that car at any given time, there would be a crumpled-up cheeseburger wrapper from her favorite drive-thru.

Terry joined a ski club and traveled the world. After every ski trip, she returned home with sore muscles and swore that next year, she was going to get in shape *before* the trip. Despite the best of intentions, her exercise bike continued to function primarily as a place to hang laundry.

Life sped by, and Terry found herself on the brink of becoming a grandmother. She retired from teaching and jumped headfirst into being a full-time nana. She missed seeing her teacher besties every day, but she continued to crack them up at frequent happy hours and book club meetings. Terry read fifty-seven books during the first year of her retirement, which gave her a tremendously larger vocabulary and lots to discuss with her friends at book club.

Some of the best days of her life were times spent with her grandson, eating Happy Meals, and sitting in her car for hours with him while he pretended to drive them to imaginary destinations.

But then it started. She couldn't find her words. Her friends at book club reassured her, "Oh, Terry. That's happening to all of us! Senior moments."

They weren't senior moments. Language was evading this quick-witted lady. First, she lost nouns. Then verbs. When Terry said, "She went there and did a hundred," she meant Diane went to the mall and spent a hundred dollars. Her family was often left to guess what she was trying to say, and frustration grew.

At age sixty-nine, she saw a specialist in memory disorders and was diagnosed with the logopenic subtype of Alzheimer's disease. The term *logopenic* comes from the Greek roots *logo*, referring to "words or speech," and *penia*, meaning "lack of." This subtype starts with significant language challenges. That's the opposite of most cases of Alzheimer's, in which memory problems start first and language problems come later.

Terry embraced the diagnosis to fight it. When first diagnosed, she still had good insight and immediately shared her diagnosis with dear friends. In a moment when her variable language challenge was not as bad, she proclaimed, "I'm the face of Alzheimer's!"

She took the disease head-on—or so she thought. Although her insight and memory centers were relatively intact, her motivation center was not.

That is something people may not know if they haven't lived with someone with Alzheimer's disease: the disease destroys the motivation center in the brain. Often, Alzheimer's patients literally cannot start something new or make a change despite the best of intentions.

Terry's neurologist recommended that she stay social, keep reading books, start exercising, and follow the Mediterranean diet.

"Yes!" she exclaimed. She would do all of these things. But she didn't because she couldn't. After a lifetime of exercising one week per year and eating convenience food, she was unable to initiate and form new habits to make these critical changes.

And so, Alzheimer's did to Terry what it does to most of its victims: it ravaged her brain. Once her language was gone, the disease stole memory and then moved on to rob her of her ability to walk. She became bedridden and dependent on full-time caregivers for her every need, which she had no way to express.

After seven years of relentless decline, her soul was released from this horrific disease that stole her personality, reduced her to a skeleton, and robbed her of every memory she held dear.

Terry was my mother.

My mom was not lazy. Nor was she overtly unhealthy. Most of her health habits were just average. As the American diet shifted from home-cooked meals to prepackaged grab-and-go microwavable meals, she shifted right along with it. She and her contemporaries were more sedentary at work than their parents' generation had been. The lifestyle conveniences that emerged in the second half of the twentieth century had hidden dangers, of which few people were fully aware.

What plagued her health were several features of the typical American lifestyle: processed food, lack of exercise, and chronic stress. And all of those increased her risk of Alzheimer's disease.

Terry was an absolute rockstar when it came to cognitive exercise. Reading fifty-seven books in one year? That's stellar. But she needed to make headway in all the lifestyle categories—nutrition, exercise, education, sleep, stress and mood, general medical health, and exposure to toxins—to have the best shot at staving off Alzheimer's disease.

If you have a lifestyle category where you excel, that's a great start. But it doesn't lessen the necessity of optimizing your other lifestyle categories.

You may have a phenomenal exercise habit, but you can't exercise away the risk that comes from terrible sleep patterns. Similarly, you can't compensate for lack of exercise by reading, and you can't sleep away the damage caused by the standard American diet's processed foods.

The best way to maximize brain health and reduce your risk of Alzheimer's disease and related dementias is to make improvements in all lifestyle areas. Strive to make progress in every area. You will be glad you did.

Take Action: Tasks, Goals, and Mini Habits

Self-assessment: Rate the following lifestyle categories using a scale from 1 to 10, where 1 is least and 10 is most.

How optimal do you think your habits are in each of the following categories?

- ☐ Nutrition _____
- ☐ Sleep _____
- ☐ Exercise _____
- ☐ Education and brain exercise _____
- ☐ General health _____
- ☐ Stress and mood _____
- ☐ Exposure to toxins _____

How motivated are you to make changes in each of the following categories?

- ☐ Nutrition _____
- ☐ Sleep _____
- ☐ Exercise _____
- ☐ Education and brain exercise _____
- ☐ General health _____

- ☐ Stress and mood _____
- ☐ Exposure to toxins _____

Map out the order you think you want to start adopting new habits in each category, where 1 is first and 7 is last

- ☐ Nutrition _____
- ☐ Sleep _____
- ☐ Exercise _____
- ☐ Education and brain exercise _____
- ☐ General health _____
- ☐ Stress and mood _____
- ☐ Exposure to toxins _____

CHAPTER 6

Nourishing Your Brain

Preventative brain health doesn't start at the doctor's office. It starts at your dinner table. What you eat and drink directly impacts your brain health.[1] Although the brain is only 2% of your body weight, it gets 15% of the blood flow from your heart and uses 20% of your body's energy. It's essential to supply your brain with the nutrients it needs to stay healthy.

Research into nutrition and brain health has exploded over the past couple of decades. We have a much better understanding of which foods benefit the brain and which foods harm it than we had in the late twentieth century.

We live in a world saturated with refined sugars, processed grains, sugary beverages, and seed oils (canola oil, vegetable oil, etc.). In the next several chapters, you'll learn how they compromise brain health and overall well-being. Before we get there, let's learn about the brain-boosting powers of the food and drink we are going to use to crowd them out: protein, fruits, vegetables, nuts, seeds, water, and tea.

Protein: Providing Critical Building Blocks

Proteins are made up of amino acids. When you eat a protein, your digestive tract disassembles it into its amino acid building blocks. Your body absorbs the amino acids, then reassembles them to build a multitude of new proteins that your body and brain need, like muscles, neurotransmitters, and antioxidants. A diet full of diverse proteins from animal or plant sources supplies your body with the extensive array of amino acids you need to thrive.

The brain uses amino acids to build brain structure and repair damaged brain tissue. Amino acids are also involved in four of the core processes of Alzheimer's disease: neurotransmitter imbalance, brain inflammation, oxidation, and beta-amyloid deposition.

There are several ways to determine if you are getting enough protein to support your health goals. The US Department of Agriculture Recommended Daily Allowance (USDA RDA) is a good place to start. The RDA is 0.36 grams of protein intake per pound that you weigh. If you don't have any medical conditions that limit your protein intake, you can multiply your weight in pounds by 0.36 to determine your bare minimum protein intake recommendation in grams.

USDA RDA for protein:
_____(weight in pounds) x 0.36 = ____ grams

Keep in mind that this is the minimum daily protein recommended to meet basic nutritional needs. If you're not sure that you're getting enough protein, track your daily food intake for several days. If you find you aren't meeting the RDA, see Appendix A for foods you could add to reach your goals. Once you are meeting the RDA, consult your healthcare provider or other trusted nutritional resource to determine your optimal daily protein intake based on your age, health goals, and medical considerations. Institute mini habits to gradually increase your protein intake toward your protein goal.

Essential Amino Acids

There are twenty amino acids. Your body uses all of them daily to assemble the proteins required for life, and you can make most of them. However, there are nine you can't make: histidine, isoleucine, leucine, methionine, phenylalanine, threonine, tryptophan, and valine. They're called essential amino acids because it's essential that you eat proteins that contain them. Foods that contain all nine essential amino acids are called "complete proteins." Meat, poultry, fish, eggs, and dairy are all complete proteins. Vegetarian complete proteins include quinoa; soy products such as tofu, tempeh, and edamame; buckwheat; chia seeds; hemp seeds; and spirulina. Phenylalanine and tryptophan are two notable essential amino acids that we'll discuss because the body needs them to build neurotransmitters.

Neurotransmitters

You'll recall from Chapter 3 that neurotransmitters are chemicals neurons use to communicate. Serotonin, a neurotransmitter known for its role in mood regulation, appetite regulation, and emotional well-being, is synthesized from the essential amino acid tryptophan. Dopamine and norepinephrine are associated with aspects of attention, pleasure, and motivation. They are derived from the essential amino acid phenylalanine. Imbalanced neurotransmitter levels impair mood and cognitive function and are associated with Alzheimer's disease.[2]

Low protein intake diminishes the availability of these essential amino acids, which impacts production of these vital neurotransmitters. People who eat more protein tend to maintain their memory and other cognitive functions better than those who eat less protein.[3] Imbalanced neurotransmitter levels impair mood and cognitive function and are associated with an increased risk of dementia.

Oxidation

Antioxidants are molecules that neutralize harmful free radicals, and many antioxidants are proteins composed of amino acids. While you absorb some antioxidants from foods, particularly fruits and vegetables, your body also manufactures crucial antioxidants from amino acids. Protein deficiency can rob the body of its ability to generate adequate antioxidant defenses. When you don't have enough antioxidants, your brain is more susceptible to oxidation.

Beta-Amyloid Buildup

Proteins fold to form three-dimensional structures. For most proteins, there is a right way and a wrong way to fold. When folded correctly, their structure allows them to function normally. When folded incorrectly, proteins can be dysfunctional and even become toxic. Unfortunately, proteins don't always fold correctly on their own. To foster correct folding, our body produces a collection of proteins called *chaperones*.

Beta-amyloid is a protein that folds. When it folds correctly, the mechanisms in our body that break it down are able to do so. When it folds incorrectly, it becomes resistant to these natural breakdown mechanisms and can build up. Chaperone proteins help beta-amyloid fold properly and assist with its breakdown.[4] Because chaperones are proteins built from amino acids, insufficient protein intake can compromise the production and function of these clearance-related proteins, leading to excess accumulation of beta-amyloid in the brain.

Plant-Based Bounty: Fruits and Vegetables

Fruits and vegetables are abundant in antioxidants, vitamins, minerals, and fiber. These natural powerhouses combat several of the core mechanisms of Alzheimer's disease.

Antioxidants

Flavonoids and polyphenols are two special groups of antioxidants found in fruits and vegetables. In their regular role as antioxidants, they soak up free radicals, reducing oxidative stress in the brain. Certain flavonoids, like those found in cocoa and blueberries, have been linked to improved blood flow to the brain. Better blood circulation can enhance cognitive function. Regular consumption of foods rich in these compounds has been associated with a lower risk of age-related cognitive decline and diseases like dementia. Fruits and vegetables rich in flavonoids and polyphenols include berries, citrus fruits, onions, kale, and spinach.

Vitamins and Minerals

Fruits and vegetables are outstanding whole-food sources of vitamins and minerals that your brain and body need to thrive. Although you can take vitamins in pill form, when you eat fruits and vegetables, you absorb additional complementary nutrients that enhance their absorption and potency. Here are a couple of brain benefits of vitamins and minerals that may surprise you: vitamin C supports neurotransmitter production, potassium helps maintain electrical activity in the nervous system, and vitamin K found in leafy green vegetables may help protect neurons from beta-amyloid.

Fiber

Fruits and vegetables provide healthy sugars that your body uses for energy. Most of the sugar in fruit is called **fructose**. Refined sugars, like glucose (listed as dextrose in processed foods) and sucrose (table sugar), are absorbed quickly, and that causes a sudden spike in blood sugar. But your body absorbs fructose more gradually, so you don't get that dramatic spike. Nature has packaged the sugars in fruit along with protective antioxidants, so you get maximum energy from them without the harmful effects of industrially refined sugars.

Fruits and vegetables are also an excellent source of dietary fiber, which is often lacking in the standard American diet. Eating fiber isn't directly about feeding the brain but rather about supporting overall health, which in turn positively impacts brain function. When you eat fiber, it stays in your gut. You don't use it for fuel, but the trillion bacteria that live in your gut do. (Yes, trillion!) In fact, these bacteria are so plentiful that there is more DNA in your body that belongs to these bugs than belongs to you! These microbes work tirelessly to maintain your health. Not only do they assist in digestion, but they also produce vitamins and support your central nervous system. Emerging research shows that a healthy gut ecosystem is associated with good mental health and improved cognitive function.

Our approach to figuring out if you are eating enough fiber is similar to our approach regarding protein. If you aren't sure you're getting enough fiber, you can consult your medical provider or nutritionist, or you can check the guidelines provided by the National Institutes of Health online. The website is listed in the "Take Action" section at the end of this chapter. Keep a food diary for several days to see how much fiber you're getting. If you are already at the recommended target or above, great! If you've got some work to do, be sure to set mini goals to increase by a modest amount of daily fiber each week—not more than 5 grams. Sudden increases in fiber intake can cause gastrointestinal distress.

Five servings of fruits and vegetables daily seems to be optimal for health.[5] Aim for two servings of fruit and three servings of vegetables daily. A few small tweaks may be all you need. Adding a handful of blueberries to your breakfast and having an apple as a snack are easy ways to add fruits. Dessert is another opportunity to enjoy a serving of fruit. Incorporating salad at lunch and another salad and serving of vegetables at dinner can help you accomplish your vegetable intake goals without much effort.

Consider Buying Organic

I used to think the emphasis on buying organic foods was nothing more than hype or marketing. However, my study of brain wellness has convinced me that we should do everything possible to avoid toxins. Unfortunately, conventionally grown foods are often treated with pesticides and herbicides that can leave toxic residues in food. Consider glyphosate, the most heavily applied weed killer in the world. In mice, laboratory studies show that glyphosate enters brain cells and drives inflammation. Specifically, glyphosate increases a harmful compound in the brain called tumor necrosis factor alpha, which plays a role in the development of Alzheimer's disease.[6]

You can reduce your exposure to toxins by eating organic foods. Organic farmers utilize natural approaches to managing pests and boosting soil fertility instead of relying on synthetic pesticides, herbicides, and fertilizers. This extra care comes at a higher price, so organic foods are more expensive than conventionally grown foods. Leveraging the Environmental Working Group's (EWG.org) research will help you get the most bang for your buck when grocery shopping. Every year, the EWG publishes their "Dirty Dozen" list of twelve fruits and vegetables that have the highest pesticide residues. They also publish a list of the fifteen that are the least contaminated with pesticides—the "Clean Fifteen." If you are able to switch some of your food purchases to organic, prioritize replacing fruits and vegetables on their Dirty list. At the time of this writing, those are strawberries, spinach, kale, grapes, peaches, pears, nectarines, apples, bell and hot peppers, cherries, blueberries, and green beans.

Nutrient-Packed Gems: Nuts and Seeds

Nuts and seeds have long been celebrated for their delicious taste, culinary utility, and exceptional nutritional value. They're loaded with compounds known to help lower the risk of dementia—omega-3 fatty acids, vitamins, minerals, and antioxidants. In our action plan, we'll embrace their salty and crunchy characteristics to crowd out nutritionally devoid snacks like potato chips and crackers.

Omega-3 Fatty Acids

Nuts are an excellent source of brain-healthy omega-3 fatty acids like alpha-linolenic acid (ALA). ALA is crucial for brain cell membrane structure and function and is linked to improved memory and mood. Walnuts, flaxseed, and chia seeds are some of the best sources of ALA.

Vitamins and Minerals

Nuts and seeds are packed with an impressive array of vitamins and minerals that promote learning and memory. Their B vitamins (notably B6, B12, and folate) help your brain produce and regulate neurotransmitters. Plus, they have minerals like copper, magnesium, and zinc that keep your nerves firing properly and the synapses between neurons functioning smoothly. Magnesium, in particular, plays a role in learning and memory.

Antioxidants

Nuts are packed with antioxidants that fight oxidative stress. Vitamin E is a powerful antioxidant that helps protect cell membranes in the brain from damage caused by free radicals. This protection may aid in preserving cognitive function as you age. Vitamin E is found abundantly in almonds and hazelnuts.

Water: The Elixir of the Brain

Water is vital for maintaining the structure, function, and overall health of the brain. Staying hydrated and drinking enough water during the day is an important step toward staying sharp. Understanding water's critical functions in the brain makes it easy to see how even mild dehydration can make it harder to focus and perform mental tasks.

Brain Shrinkage

Because the brain is more than 70% water, dehydration can temporarily shrink it. This shrinkage affects brain function, leading to difficulties in reasoning, problem-solving, and decision-making. As we age, our thirst sensation decreases.[7] Seniors can get dehydrated without feeling thirsty. They also have a lower percentage of total body water. These two factors make seniors more likely to develop symptomatic dehydration, which can lead to confusion and necessitate emergency room visits.

Brain Protection

Water also supports the brain's health by cushioning it. The brain and spinal cord are surrounded by cerebrospinal fluid (CSF), which is 99% water; the other 1% is made up of proteins, ions, and glucose. CSF acts as a shock absorber, protecting the brain from sudden jolts. The brain makes about 16 ounces of CSF daily. Making sure you're well-hydrated allows your brain to continue making this essential fluid.

Transport Systems

Staying hydrated also allows for nutrient delivery and waste removal. Water transports essential nutrients and oxygen in the bloodstream. Proper hydration ensures these vital elements reach the brain cells and nourish them. After delivering its nutrients, water flushes waste out of brain cells and carries it away. This process maintains a clean and healthy environment for brain cells to function well. Dehydration interferes with nutrient delivery and waste-removal systems. Lack of nutrients puts neurons on the path toward a cellular energy crisis. Without enough water to take out the cellular garbage, harmful substances build up in neurons and can impair brain performance.

Electrolytes

Water also helps maintain the delicate balance of electrolytes (like sodium, chloride, and potassium) necessary for proper nerve signaling. An imbalance causes slower and less efficient communication between neurons, leading to delays in processing information, slower reaction times, and decreased overall mental agility.

Tea: The Steeped Solution for Brainpower

Drinking tea is a great way to crowd out sugary beverages while nurturing brain health and promoting mental clarity. Although white tea, black tea, and oolong tea all contain antioxidants and other brain-benefiting compounds, green tea tends to offer more pronounced brain benefits compared to other types of tea primarily because of its higher concentration of certain beneficial compounds, particularly epigallocatechin gallate (EGCG) and L-theanine.

EGCG is a potent antioxidant that's plentiful in green tea and offers remarkable brain health benefits. In addition to reducing oxidative stress and inflammation in the brain, EGCG also promotes the growth of new neurons and enhances brain connectivity. Studies reveal that regular consumption of EGCG-rich green tea has been associated with improved cognitive abilities.[8]

L-theanine is a compound found in green tea that is derived from the amino acid glutamine. It's known for its calming effect on the brain. L-theanine promotes alpha-wave activity, which is an interesting state for the brain to be in. When your brain is making alpha waves, you'll feel relaxed and tranquil but not drowsy. You'll also have great focus and creativity. In addition, L-theanine modulates neurotransmitters, like dopamine and serotonin, improving mood and reducing stress and anxiety levels. Overall, L-theanine's ability to promote relaxation without sedation, coupled with its positive impact on cognitive function, makes it a valuable compound in supporting brain health.

A Final Word on Food Choice

As you work to increase your intake of the foods mentioned in this chapter, choose natural, whole foods or minimally processed foods to reach your goals. Industrial food technology has made food less expensive and easier to consume, but the convenience comes with a price in terms of brain health.

Ultra-processed foods (UPFs) have been heavily altered in factories. We identify many UPFs as junk food, such as cheese puffs, fast-food, frozen pizza, sugary cereal, and pastries. But there are many UPFs masquerading as healthy foods—items like energy drinks, breakfast bars, low-fat coffee creamers, flavored yogurts, and hummus. You can identify UPFs by their long list of ingredients. If you need a degree in chemistry to understand the contents, that food is likely a UPF. They often have a long shelf life, indicating that they contain chemical preservatives. UPFs have become a staple of the US diet, even though they have fewer nutrients than whole foods and are often loaded with refined sugar, seed oils, artificial additives, and preservatives. These foods have a negative impact on brain health. Researchers have reported a link between high consumption of UPFs and cognitive decline.[9]

The NOVA Group's Open Food Facts website is an excellent resource for learning more about identifying and avoiding UPFs: https://world.openfoodfacts.org/nova. In addition to information, they offer a free mobile app that allows you to scan food barcodes and returns a score that indicates how processed it is. It can be a valuable tool in helping you choose less-processed foods at the grocery store.

Take Action: Tasks, Goals, and Mini Habits

Eat a diet rich in nourishing proteins that your brain and body need

- ☐ Determine your RDA minimum daily intake for protein (in grams). Either multiply your weight in pounds by 0.36, use the USDA protein calculator at https://www.nal.usda.gov/human-nutrition-and-food-safety/dri-calculator, or refer to the National Institutes of Health Daily Reference Intakes for Macronutrients and Water: https://www.ncbi.nlm.nih.gov/books/NBK56068/table/summarytables.t4.

- ☐ Keep a daily food diary for a week to track your protein intake. Refer to Appendix A, nutrition labels, and online nutrition trackers to determine the protein content of your meals and snacks.

- [ ] If your daily intake is below the RDA, set mini habits to increase daily protein intake by 5 grams each week until you reach the RDA.
- [ ] Once you are meeting the recommended daily intake of protein, consult your physician to determine your optimal daily protein intake, considering your age, health goals, and medical concerns.
- [ ] Increase your daily protein intake by 5 grams each week until you reach your optimal protein amount.

Eat a variety of fruits and vegetables to obtain a broad range of the nutrients and fiber that are essential for maintaining a healthy brain

- [ ] Tally the servings of fruits and vegetables you ate yesterday and today. If you aren't getting 5 servings most days, set up your weekly mini habits to increase intake:
  - Add an easy morning fruit snack every day for a week—like an apple, orange, or banana.
  - Add a serving of fruit to your breakfast. Or, if you have an egg-based savory breakfast, add a serving of vegetables to your scramble.
  - Add salad to your lunch.
  - Add an easy afternoon vegetable snack—like carrots or celery sticks.
  - Add salad to your dinner.

BRAIN HEALTH ACTION PLAN

- o Add a serving of raw or cooked vegetables to your dinner.
- o If you eat dessert, have a serving of fruit for dessert one night per week.
  - ☐ Increase the number of fruit desserts you eat weekly until you have crowded out most processed non-fruit desserts that contain high amounts of added sugar.
  - ☐ Determine your recommended daily fiber intake. A useful table is available at https://www.ncbi.nlm.nih.gov/books/NBK56068/table/summarytables.t4.
  - ☐ Review your fruit and vegetable intake as well as grain and nut intake to ensure that you are getting adequate fiber. Five servings of vegetables are usually enough, but if you find the types you are eating don't get you to your fiber target, gradually increase fiber with mini habits.
- o Add a serving of food that contains 5 grams of fiber daily for one week.
- o Continue to add a daily serving of fiber (5 grams) each week until you meet your goal.

Decrease your intake of ultra-processed foods

- ☐ Visit https://world.openfoodfacts.org/nova for more information about processed foods.

- ☐ Consider downloading the NOVA Group's free mobile app, Open Food Facts. It allows you to scan foods and rates them from 1 to 4 based on how processed they are, with 4 meaning it's a UPF.
- ☐ Decrease the number of UPFs that come into your home. Each week, use the app to scan the foods you are considering buying in one aisle of your grocery shopping trip. Try to replace one level-4 UPF with an alternative that is a level 2 or 3. The goal is to decrease the number of 4s you purchase. It's nearly impossible to cut them out completely. Once you have finished the aisles, spend the next three weeks scanning the items on each wall of the perimeter of the grocery store.

Reap the health benefits of nuts and seeds

- ☐ Shop for nuts and seeds. Read labels to be sure they aren't roasted in seed oils: canola oil (rapeseed), corn oil, sesame oil, safflower oil, cottonseed oil, and soybean oil. (We'll cover why in Chapter 8.)
- ☐ Add a serving of nuts or seeds to your salads.
- ☐ Plan ahead. Portion nuts or homemade trail mix into resealable bags that you can keep with you throughout the day to help redirect you away from processed snacks when you are craving salt or crunch.

Drink adequate water for optimal brain health

Determine your optimal water intake: 8 glasses (64 ounces or a half gallon) is a standard goal if you don't have any medical concerns that limit water intake.

- ☐ Purchase a reusable water bottle that holds enough water for your day's intake goal. Fill it every morning and keep it with you throughout the day to keep you on track. This can be a bottle of water from the grocery store or a reusable jug that has times marked off to help you gradually meet your hydration goals throughout the day.

- ☐ If you get to the evening and haven't met your goal, do not try to catch up at that point. You might derail deep sleep with numerous bathroom visits. Fill your bottle and commit to getting closer to your goal the next day.

Drink green tea for its brain-boosting compounds

- ☐ Purchase appealing varieties of green tea—caffeinated and/or decaffeinated, depending on when you plan to work them into your schedule.

- ☐ Add 1 cup of decaffeinated green tea each evening after dinner.

- ☐ Add 1 cup of green tea either in the morning or the afternoon.

Notes

[1] Gustavo Díaz, Laetitia Lengele, Sandrine Sourdet, Gaëlle Soriano, and Philipe de Souto Barreto, "Nutrients and amyloid β status in the brain: A narrative review," Ageing Res Rev 81 (November 2022):101728, https://doi.org/10.1016/j.arr.2022.101728.

[2] Stuart G. Snowden et al., "Neurotransmitter Imbalance in the Brain and Alzheimer's Disease Pathology," Journal of Alzheimer's disease 72, no. 1 (2019): 35–43, https://doi.org/10.3233/JAD-190577.

[3] Tian-Shin Yeh, Changzheng Yuan, Alberto Ascherio, et al., "Long-term dietary protein intake and subjective cognitive decline in US men and women," Am J Clin Nutr. 115, no. 1 (2022):199–210, https://doi.org/10.1093%2Fajcn%2Fnqab236.

[4] Zaida L. Almeida and Rui M. M. Brito, "Amyloid Disassembly: What Can We Learn from Chaperones?" Biomedicines 10, no. 12 (December 2022):3276, https://doi.org/10.3390/biomedicines10123276.

[5] Dong D. Wang, Yanping Li, et al., "Fruit and Vegetable Intake and Mortality: Results From 2 Prospective Cohort Studies of US Men and Women and a Meta-Analysis of 26 Cohort Studies," Circulation 143, no. 17 (April 2021):1642–1654, https://doi.org/10.1161/circulationaha.120.048996.

[6] Joanna K. Winstone, Khyatiben V. Pathak, Wendy Winslow, Ignazio S. Piras, Jennifer White, Ritin Sharma, Matthew J. Huentelman, Patrick Pirrotte, and Ramon Velazquez, "Glyphosate infiltrates the brain and increases pro-inflammatory cytokine TNFα: implications for neurodegenerative disorders," J Neuroinflammation 19, no. 193 (July 2022), https://doi.org/10.1186/s12974-022-02544-5.

[7] B. J. Rolls and P. A. Phillips, "Aging and disturbances of thirst and fluid balance," Nutrition reviews 48, no. 3 (1990):137–44, https://doi.org/10.1111/j.1753-4887.1990.tb02915.x

[8] Yoshitake Baba, Shun Inagaki, Sae Nakagawa, et al., "Effect of Daily Intake of Green Tea Catechins on Cognitive Function in Middle-Aged and Older Subjects: A Randomized, Placebo-Controlled Study," Molecules 25, no. 18 (September 2020):4265, https://doi.org/10.3390/molecules25184265.

[9] Natalia Gomes Gonçalves, Naomi Vidal Ferreira, Neha Khandpur, et al., "Association Between Consumption of Ultraprocessed Foods and Cognitive Decline," JAMA Neurol. 80, no. 2 (2023):142–150, https://doi.org/10.1001/jamaneurol.2022.4397.

CHAPTER 7

Sugar, Sweet Saboteur

Sugar Addict? I've Been There.

You will probably be shocked to hear that there was a Starbucks across the street from my office. (Shocked that there was only one, that is!) Anyway, I developed quite a chai latte habit. Having a chai latte before work was a given. It wasn't long before I ramped up to include a second latte during my midmorning break. Heavy afternoon eyes often told my legs to take a third trip across the street.

On my days off, I had a similar pattern. Finding myself five minutes early to pick up my daughter from violin practice, I'd think, *Why not make good use of this time and treat myself to a chai latte?* The honest answer would have been, "Because it doesn't take five minutes to run into Starbucks. It takes ten." I ignored that reality and continued to indulge at every opportunity. The sight of my occupied cup holder induced shame as I arrived late to find my daughter standing patiently on the sidewalk after her lesson. This pattern repeated daily because there is a

Starbucks on the way to every errand, meeting, and pickup. I sabotaged my schedule constantly. I inconvenienced my family and everyone who was expecting me to be on time, and I felt terrible about it. But I kept it up. This is addiction behavior. I was addicted to sugar, and chai lattes were the ever-present vehicle to feed my addiction.

A grande chai latte has 24 grams of added sugar. In lattes alone, I was racking up 72 grams of added sugar most days! Combine that with the added sugar in the rest of the food I was eating daily without being mindful of the nutrition labels (a cup of vanilla yogurt here and some cookies there), and I was consistently eating over 100 grams of added sugar daily. I didn't recognize my addiction until I saw the movie *Fed Up* with my family. This movie opened my eyes. I highly recommend watching it.

That's when I took steps to change this habit. If I can get from over 100 grams of added sugar daily to a more reasonable 20 to 30 added grams daily, I'm confident you can too.

This chapter will help you understand how sugar contributes to Alzheimer's disease, how to set a healthy sugar-intake goal, and the steps to achieve that goal with less struggle than you might expect.

Sugar Causes Brain Disease

The steady rise in the consumption of added sugars is a defining characteristic of the modern American diet. Not only is sugar driving the obesity epidemic, it's at the heart of brain disease.

Sugar increases toxic protein in the brain, disrupts neurotransmitter balance, fosters inflammation, promotes oxidative stress, damages blood vessels, and fuels addictive behaviors—collectively increasing the risk of Alzheimer's disease. In short, it revs up every core process of Alzheimer's disease.

The standard American diet is full of processed, high-sugar foods. The rapid and excessive consumption of sugar leads to erratic spikes and crashes in blood sugar levels, initiating a cascade of effects that harm the brain. When you eat food with added sugar, you get a big spike in your blood sugar. Your body responds by releasing a big dose of insulin to push that glucose into your cells, where it can be used as fuel to create energy.

> *High glycemic index foods produce a rapid, sharp spike in blood sugar levels, while low glycemic index foods result in a more gradual and lower blood sugar peak.*

After insulin has done its job, it must be broken down (degraded) before your body clears it. The enzyme that breaks down insulin is called insulin-degrading enzyme (IDE). Although that sounds straightforward, when scientists named that enzyme, they didn't know that it breaks down other proteins as well. As it turns out, IDE also breaks down beta-amyloid, one of the toxic proteins associated with Alzheimer's disease. That means that insulin and beta-amyloid compete to get broken down by IDE, but insulin has a competitive advantage due to its smaller size. So when your system is exposed to high sugar levels, IDE tends to prioritize breaking down insulin. That leads to elevated beta-amyloid levels in the bloodstream. This has devastating consequences: the beta-amyloid that doesn't get broken down can end up being stored in the brain.

> **The glycemic index** (GI) ranks foods according to how quickly they raise blood sugar. High glycemic index foods produce a rapid, sharp spike in blood sugar levels, while low glycemic index foods result in a more gradual and lower blood sugar peak.

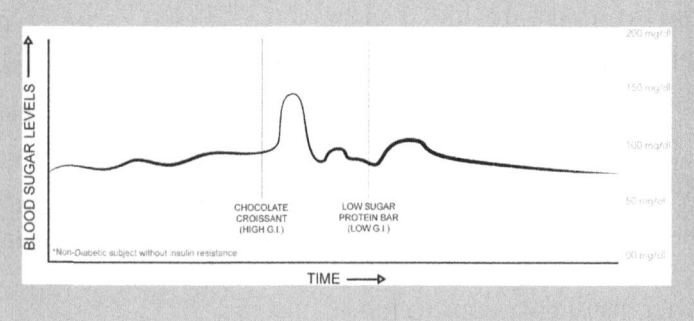

Sugar is addictive.[1] This adds another layer of complexity to its harmful effects on the brain. Like other addictive substances, sugar triggers the brain's reward system to release the neurotransmitter dopamine. Dopamine creates the pleasurable feeling of the sugar high and reinforces the desire for more sugar. The cycle of reward and craving overpowers our will and keeps us overconsuming sugar. And the neurotransmitter story gets worse. As we've discussed, the body is flooded with insulin in response to surging blood sugar levels. Insulin works to decrease blood sugar, but insulin also abruptly drops dopamine levels, quickly taking the brain from a high dopamine state to a low dopamine state. That causes mood swings and lack of motivation. It can even impair thinking—all the familiar feelings of the sugar crash.

Chronic consumption of high-sugar foods is linked to increased inflammation throughout the body and brain. The inflammatory response triggered by excess sugar intake works in the typical way described in Chapter 3: by damaging the protective blood-brain barrier and allowing toxins and inflammatory molecules to infiltrate the brain.

Sugar's negative impact on the brain also includes oxidative stress. Understand that, when faced with a sugar spike, every part of the body works to get rid of it as quickly as possible. It's like a game of hot potato. When you eat high-sugar foods, your gut rapidly absorbs sugar and transfers it to your bloodstream. High sugar in your bloodstream triggers the swift release of insulin to alleviate high blood sugar by prompting your cells to absorb the sugar. Your cells can't transfer the sugar out. The only way the cells can get rid of the sugar is to ramp up metabolism to burn the sugar and generate energy. Although producing extra energy might sound appealing, the energy produced that is beyond our metabolic needs get stored as fat. You'll recall from Chapter 3 that the process of metabolizing sugar generates unstable free radicals that can damage brain cells. Loading the system with sugar pushes cell metabolism into overdrive, generating more free radicals than the brain's antioxidant defenses can neutralize. This oxidative stress can lead to brain cell dysfunction and cell death, which accelerates brain aging. The diagram below illustrates how high sugar creates oxidative stress at a cellular level.

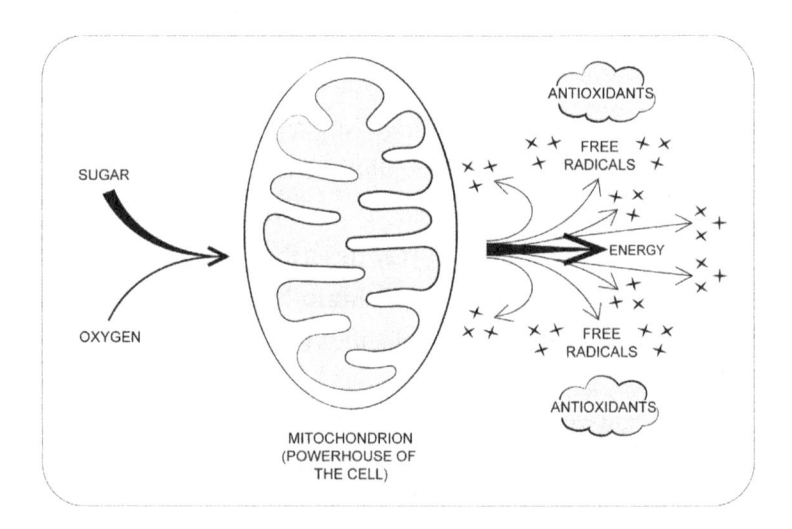

Acknowledging the profound influence of sugar on brain health is the first step toward mindfully reevaluating dietary habits to stave off Alzheimer's disease.

The Scope of the Sugar Problem

The average American consumes 70 grams—about 17 teaspoons—of added sugar daily. Put another way, that's over a pound of added sugar per week! Most of us aren't adding 17 teaspoons of sugar to our morning coffee, so how is all of this sugar getting into our system?

The fact is, added sugar is everywhere. It's almost impossible to find processed food that doesn't have sugar or high fructose corn syrup toward the top of the ingredient list. You expect to find added sugars in cakes, cookies, and sugary cereals. But you might not expect to find added sugars hiding in soup, whole wheat bread, granola, crackers, peanut butter, and protein bars. A slice of wheat bread can have as much added sugar as an Oreo cookie! Those unexpected places are great targets for slashing sugar without missing it.

Before you get too overwhelmed, understand that completely eliminating all added sugar is not our goal. Moderation and making healthy choices that satisfy our cravings and offer better nutritional value are our goals. I follow the **American Heart Association (AHA) guidelines** for added sugar. The AHA recommends no more than 25 grams (6 teaspoons) of added sugar daily for women and 36 grams (9 teaspoons) of added sugar daily for men. Sorry, ladies.

Reading labels is a must. The nutrition label is the only part of food packaging that doesn't lie, and it's the only way to find stealthily added sugars. The examples of high-added-sugar foods listed in this chapter are not unique. When you read labels, you will also find astonishing amounts of added sugar where you least expect it. Keep the AHA recommendations in mind when you buy groceries, and try to find options with no or low added sugar. Be particularly cautious about adding "reduced fat" foods to your cart without examining the nutrition label. When food manufacturers create "diet foods" by taking the fat out, they often restore flavor with sugar. Going through the cracker aisle at the grocery store, I found several brands in which the "reduced fat" or "whole wheat" version had twice the added sugar as the original cracker.

We used to be able to just "shop the walls of the grocery store" to avoid processed foods. Typically, that means the bakery, meat, deli, dairy, and produce sections. Now, even the outer sections of the grocery store are packed with processed foods containing added sugar. Processed meats, coffee creamers, and flavored yogurts are common sources of added sugar. Even the produce section isn't spared: prepared salads can have surprising amounts of added sugar. These days, it's just as important to read labels on the outer walls of the grocery store as it is in the aisles.

Some of the steps in the "Take Action" section at the end of this chapter include systematically going through your refrigerator and pantry and looking for foods that have more sugar than you expected. We'll put those aside and then head to the grocery store to find lower-sugar replacements.

Reading labels on everything you buy can seem daunting. Once you find new favorites that fit into your sugar goals, you can keep those on repeat. You'll have to read the labels only on new foods you consider.

> **"But whole fruits and vegetables don't have nutrition labels."**
>
> Right! These are some foods that give us a break from our grocery store label-reading! Whole fruits and vegetables don't have added sugar or nutrition labels, so you don't need to count them when you are tracking added sugar. Whole fruit contains a balance of glucose and fructose, some of which is bound to fiber. The balance of sugars and the fiber binding cause sugar to be released more gradually into the bloodstream, thus producing a lower blood sugar peak and a less pronounced insulin response. The process of turning fruit into juice, jam, or jelly, for example, separates fruit's natural sugars from fiber. Adding sugar is often part of the process as well. Any time fresh fruit is processed into something else, it gets a nutrition label, and the added sugar must be counted in your daily tally.

Slashing Sugar

If you read labels and are mindful about added sugar, you can follow the AHA guidelines without giving up your favorite sweet treat. By adopting a few lasting habits, you can greatly reduce sugar in places where you won't miss it and enjoy a bit of sugar in the places where it is more pleasurable. By cutting sugar out of foods that aren't sweet and aren't treats, you make room for a sweet here and there.

From breakfast to dinner, drinks to desserts, and grocery store to pantry, let's look at some of the places where added sugar is hiding so we can crowd it out.

> *Having a sweet tooth is in our DNA. It is just our craving for fruit. When our ancient ancestors craved sweets, they were driven to find fruits. Do the same. When you crave something sweet, look for fruit; it will usually satisfy you. It's amazing how much easier it becomes to phase out processed sweets like candy and cookies when you focus on attaining the health benefits of the vital compounds in fruits.*

Juicy Target: Sweetened Beverages

Sugary beverages are the number-one source of added sugar in the American diet. Sugary drinks bombard the body's system with calories, but they don't make us feel full, so they lead us to overconsume sugar. Worse, their sugars are not bound to fiber that slows their absorption. They rapidly flood the bloodstream with sugar, which, as we know, is soon followed by a flood of insulin. Animal studies show that sugar in liquid form, such as in soft drinks and juice, causes inflammation in the hippocampus, with an associated decline in short-term memory.[2]

Research on humans shows similar results. A 2017 study[3] noted that people who drank more sugary drinks had smaller brain volumes and performed worse on memory testing than people who had minimal sugary drink intake. This finding was not restricted to soft drinks. People who drank juice daily also had smaller brain volumes, including smaller hippocampal memory structures.

Fruit Juice

If you drink fruit juice, consider crowding it out by eating the whole fruit instead. Here's why: an orange contains 12 grams of natural sugar and 2.8 grams of fiber, while a glass of no-sugar-added orange juice contains 23 grams of natural sugar and no measurable fiber. The large dose of sugar in juice is absorbed more quickly than sugar from the whole fruit since it has no attached fiber to slow down its digestion. When a diabetic needs sugar, they are given orange juice, not an orange, because they need rapid access to sugar in their bloodstream. However, this is not what we want on a daily basis. The natural sugars in juice affect your system much like added sugars do, so count them in your added-sugar grams when you are tracking your daily intake.

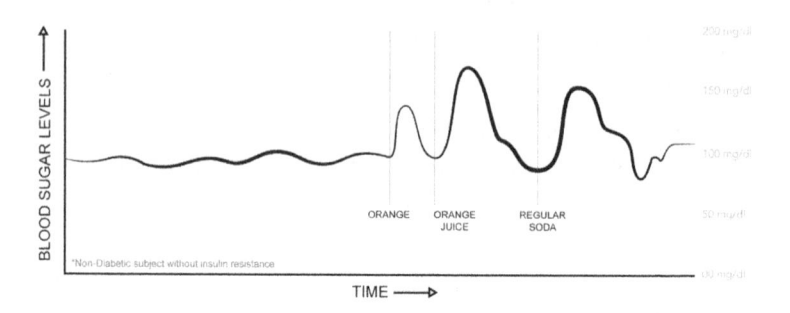

Oh, Those Fancy Coffees

Coffeehouse drinks are not exempt from your daily sugar count. In fact, this is another great place to reduce added sugar. Although Americans are drinking fewer soft drinks than in the past decades, most people have added that sugar right back in the form of daily sugar-laden coffee drinks. Most flavored coffees are sugar bombs that sabotage our health goals. It's virtually impossible to cut enough sugar out of other areas to have these indulgences daily. If you haven't perused the nutrition guide from your favorite coffee spot, you might be surprised to see just how much added sugar these drinks contain. Here are some values from the nutrition guide of a popular coffeehouse chain:

Drink	Added sugar
Medium chai latte	24 g
Medium mocha	17 g
Medium white chocolate mocha	35 g
Medium pumpkin spice latte	32 g
Medium caramel blended iced coffee	36 g

You may be thinking, *Does this mean I can't have my daily white mocha?*

In a word: yes. Sugar-filled coffees are a treat and should be thought of as a dessert. It's okay to mindfully enjoy an indulgence here and there, but as you focus on cultivating brain-healthy eating habits, you want to break the streak of *habitual* indulgence. It's not that you can never have fancy coffees. It's that you should make an effort to not have them daily. This way, when you do have them, you can fully appreciate them as the treat they are.

Put another way, consider that a white chocolate mocha has nearly the same added sugar as a McDonald's hot fudge sundae (36 grams). We wouldn't dream of having a daily morning hot fudge sundae, and yet, these coffees have snuck into our lives, offering something quite similar. While this harsh news may be hard to swallow, eating a low-sugar diet is critically important to optimizing brain health, and that's why you're reading this book.

One option is to have your mocha once a week, appreciate it for the treat it is, and have no other added sugars that day. That way, it won't derail your sugar goals too much. It could also be helpful to explore what you really like about that mocha. For me and my chai lattes, the answers were that they're warm, social, an indulgence, and full of fall spices. Most of those characteristics can be found in regular chai-flavored tea from a tea bag. A mocha is similar but with coffee and chocolate flavors. You can satisfy most of your cravings by having a coffee with unsweetened nondairy milk and a piece of chocolate to minimize overall dietary sugar. (A small latte with almond milk has 6.7 grams of sugar, and a square of dark chocolate has fewer than 4 grams of added sugar.) If you find that you use fancy coffees to reward yourself, see if you can find a nonfood reward instead.

Starting the Day with Dessert

A quarter of our daily-added-sugar intake comes from breakfast. Muffins, pastries, granola, protein drinks, and flavored yogurts can be brimming with sugar. Until I started reading labels, I had no idea that my favorite chai protein drink had nearly as much added sugar (23 grams per cup) as my favorite vanilla ice cream (27 grams per cup). Consider the chart below. While we might assume that a blueberry muffin has less added sugar than two Ding Dongs, granola has less added sugar than sugary cereals, yogurt has less added sugar than donuts, and wheat bread has less added sugar than English muffins, nutrition labels tell a different story. Here are some examples that I found at my local grocery store:

Item	Serving size	Added sugar
Blueberry muffin	3.75 oz.	33 g
Ding Dong	2 Ding Dongs	30 g
Granola	1 C	18 g
Sugary cereal	1 C	12 g
Vanilla yogurt	6 oz	14 g
Little powdered sugar donuts	3 donuts	14 g
Wheat bread	1 slice	5 g
English muffin	2 halves	0 g

Build a better breakfast. Get a jump start on achieving your protein intake goals for the day by having a high-protein breakfast. Eggs, breakfast meats, and plain Greek yogurt are high-protein foods that can crowd out sugar-loaded choices. Some of my favorite low-effort and make-ahead recipes are included in Chapter 17.

When you need a break from eggs, use the following substitutions:

Replace these:	With these:
High added sugar	Low-sugar choice
Flavored yogurt	Plain Greek yogurt with no added sugar or chia pudding (see recipes); add a handful of berries and nuts/seeds/toasted unsweetened coconut flakes/homemade granola for flavor and crunch
Store-bought granola	Make your own (see recipes)

Cereal	Buy oatmeal and cereals with no added sugar
Wheat toast	Sourdough toast, no-sugar-added English muffins

Added Sugar in Sauces and Salad Dressings

Salad Dressings

Eating more salads is a great way to increase your veggie intake. However, that usually means eating more salad dressing, which can increase added sugar intake. The amount of added sugar in dressings varies widely, so be sure to read labels and opt for the lowest-added-sugar option. Before you evaluate salad dressings, read Chapter 8 on seed oils (canola oil, vegetable oil, safflower oil, etc.), which are also often in dressings and are best avoided. There are several brands of salad dressings that are free of sugar and seed oils. You might also consider making your own dressings using natural ingredients like olive oil, vinegar, herbs, and spices. That allows you to control the ingredients and reduce or eliminate sugar. I've provided several of my favorite easy and tasty dressings in the recipe section. Making a weekly salad dressing is a great healthy habit.

Ketchup and Barbecue Sauce

These may require a bit of compromise. There are some pretty tasty low-sugar barbecue sauces to use when you're cooking at home. When you're dining out, you don't have much control over the ingredients, and restaurant barbecue sauces are likely to have high added sugar. In that situation, the best strategy for decreasing the added sugar is to limit your portion size. I recommend a similar approach for ketchup. It's chock-full of sugar, which is where most of its flavor comes from. If you are one of the many people who don't enjoy the low-sugar alternatives, opt for foods that don't require ketchup as an accompaniment. When you do have ketchup, be mindful about how much you're eating.

Snacks

Snacks are a great way to add nutrients that crowd out sources of added sugar. Whether you crave a sweet snack or a salty one, both present an opportunity to cut sugar.

Sweet Snacks

We cross paths with sweet snacks like granola bars, candies, cookies, and gummy fruit snacks throughout our day. Whether it's being offered cookies and muffins at work meetings or having to walk past twenty feet of candy displays to check out at the hardware store, processed sweets seem to be available everywhere. The best way to avoid them is to prepare healthy sweet snacks ahead of time. Fresh fruit is one of the healthiest and easiest choices. One solution is to plan two fresh fruit snacks that you can carry with you during the day. This way, when you are tempted by processed sweet snacks, you'll already have a healthier choice at your fingertips.

Salty Snacks

Salty snacks like crackers, pretzels, and chips can have unexpected added sugar, making them another great place to cut added sugar without missing it. Read labels and choose brands with lower or no added sugar. Another strategy for avoiding sugar-added salty snacks is to crowd them out with nutrient-packed nuts.

Desserts

Dessert shouldn't be a daily event. If you have a daily dessert habit, I recommend crowding out most desserts with fruit. On occasions when you do indulge in a non-fruit dessert, be aware of portion size. Many of us have become accustomed to outrageously large desserts that restaurants serve.

When reading labels, note the serving size to guide your portions. For example, my favorite vanilla ice cream specifies that a serving size is 2/3 cup and that there are 25 grams of added sugars. Enjoying ½ cup of ice cream keeps the added sugar at 18 grams, which can fit into the AHA guidelines. If ½ cup of ice cream seems too small4 for dessert, consider adding fresh or frozen fruit to increase the portion size without defeating your added-sugar goals.

Vitamins

Regrettably, chewable vitamins and vitamin drink packets often have added sugar. Read their labels and count them in your sugar totals. Ask your health provider to recommend sugar-free alternatives if you cannot swallow vitamin tablets or capsules.

Final Word: Sweeteners and Sugar Substitutes

Unfortunately, synthetic sugar substitutes are not your ally in the battle to optimize brain health by decreasing sugar intake. True, sugar substitutes can provide sweetness while avoiding the attributes of sugar that are directly linked to the core processes of Alzheimer's disease. However, the main problem with sugar substitutes is that they will not help you break your sweetness addiction. Most sugar substitutes are sweeter than cane sugar. The exaggerated sweetness profile of sugar substitutes keeps your palate accustomed to high sweetness levels. Their high sweetness hit is also shorter-lived than that which we experience from cane sugar. The brief, super-sweet high increases sweetness-seeking behavior; you will most likely end up consuming added sugar at some point in your quest to alleviate the craving.

Tricking your body with synthetic food substitutes is not the way to achieve good health. As you decrease sugar intake and avoid sugar substitutes, your palate will lose most of its habituation to sweetness and turn back into a palate satisfied with savory tastes. Later, when you come across processed sweets, you will likely find them to be overly sweet, lacking in flavor, and unsatisfying. When you get to this point, congratulations are in order. Your palate has normalized!

When you do need to add sweetness to a food or drink, opt for natural choices that have a lower glycemic index than cane sugar. Coconut sugar, honey, and maple syrup all fit the bill. They also contain trace vitamins, minerals, and antioxidants. Coconut sugar is unique in that it also contains some fiber, which slows its absorption, making it the lowest GI choice among the three.

Take Action: Tasks, Goals, and Mini Habits

Shift sugar intake to gradually get to the American Heart Association guidelines for daily added sugar.

Assess your sugar intake

- ☐ For the next week, keep a food diary on your phone. Include grams of added sugar in all the foods you eat. If you eat out, use online sources to determine the added sugar content.
    - o Total added sugars consumed day 1_____
    - o Total added sugars consumed day 2_____
    - o Total added sugars consumed day 3_____

BRAIN HEALTH ACTION PLAN

- ○ Total added sugars consumed day 4_____
- ○ Total added sugars consumed day 5_____
- ○ Total added sugars consumed day 6_____
- ○ Total added sugars consumed day 7_____
- ○ What were some surprisingly high-added-sugar foods? _____

☐ Research how much added sugar your favorite treats contain so you can see how they will fit into your goals:
  - ○ Sweet:_____ Grams added sugar:_____
  - ○ Sweet:_____ Grams added sugar:_____
  - ○ Sweet:_____ Grams added sugar:_____
  - ○ Sweet:_____ Grams added sugar:_____

Perform a pantry and refrigerator/freezer audit

(You will also do a pantry and refrigerator audit at the end of Chapter 8. Before starting your audit for added sugar, you may want to read that chapter and then decide if you'll do one combined audit for sugar and seed oils or keep them separate.)

☐ Read the labels on the items in your pantry and refrigerator. Miniaturize the goal by addressing a different shelf or food category each day or each week. If you decide to go by categories, the following list can help guide you:

☐ Pantry

- Crackers, chips, and nuts
- Cookies and candies
- Cereal, granola, granola bars, and protein bars
- Pasta sauce, salsa, and other sauces
- Peanut butter, other nut butters, and chocolate hazelnut spread
- Bread and tortillas
- Remaining items

☐ Refrigerator
- Salad dressings, marinades, and pickles
- Sauces and condiments, including ketchup and barbecue sauce
- Dairy, especially flavored milk and coffee creamers
- Jellies, jams, and flavored yogurts
- Everything in the deli drawer, including deli meats
- Any item in your veggie drawer that has a nutrition label

☐ Freezer audit: same process
- Frozen meals and frozen pizza
- Breakfast items, including breakfast sausages
- Frozen fruit (some have added sugar)
- Desserts and ice creams (Yes, they all have added sugar, but the amount can vary.

Some ice creams have 17 grams of sugar per serving, while others have 50 grams. Some brands and flavors are more likely to fit into your health goals than others.)

☐ Identify sweet items that have more than 6 grams of added sugar per serving; circle the nutrition panel with a marker.

☐ Identify savory items that have more than 2 grams of added sugar per serving (for example, crackers or bread); circle the nutrition panel with a marker.

☐ When you finish an item with a circled nutrition label, take a picture of the item and nutrition label with your phone.

☐ Make an album of these items and their nutrition labels on your phone.

☐ Find lower-sugar alternatives to replace them the next time you buy groceries.

De-sugar your breakfast

☐ Plan savory, high-protein-centered breakfasts.*

☐ Swap out flavored yogurt for plain Greek yogurt or chia pudding* with fresh or frozen (no added sugar) fruit.

☐ Swap out added-sugar cereal and granola for no-sugar-added options, or make granola* or overnight oats.*

☐ Swap out breakfast baked goods like muffins, banana bread, and pastries for baked oats.*

☐ Swap out wheat toast for zero-added sugar sourdough toast or English muffins.

☐ Replace any fruit juice you drink with water and eat the whole fruit instead.

*See Chapter 17 for recipes.

Crowd out sweet temptations with fruit

☐ Stock up on fresh fruit for the week; prep and package it into servings if necessary.

☐ Keep fruit snacks with you to crowd out tempting snacks that have added sugar or to use as an interruption when a craving for a sweet arises.

Don't drink sugar, part one: cold beverages

☐ Read labels on everything cold that you drink; set aside those with added sugar.

☐ Eat fresh fruit instead of drinking fruit juice.

☐ Crowd out energy drinks and regular and diet soda (decrease by one drink per day, per week) with water, water with a squeeze of citrus, mineral water, or flavored seltzer with no added sugar or artificial sweeteners.

☐ Crowd out sweetened tea with unsweetened tea.

Don't drink sugar, part two: hot beverages

- ☐ Assess the sugar in your hot beverages.

- ☐ If you sweeten coffee or tea at home, aim to decrease to ½ teaspoon of sugar (that's 2 grams of sugar, which is likely to fit into your AHA daily-added-sugar goal).

- ☐ If you use coffee creamer, check the label for added sugars, and check the level of processing on the Open Food Facts app (discussed in Chapter 6). Crowd out with lower-sugar, less-processed options, such as unsweetened cream, half-and-half, milk, nut milk, or coconut milk.

- ☐ Coffee and tea elsewhere: Find out how much added sugar your favorite sweet drink has. If that information is not available at the coffeehouse, search for a similar drink on a coffeehouse chain's website and write the amount here: ____grams

- ☐ Determine how often you will have that high-sugar coffee drink for a treat, and minimize sugar intake the rest of the day: ____Once a week ____Twice a week ____Every other week ____Other

- ☐ Find suitable lower-sugar replacements for your sweet hot drink from the suggestions earlier in this chapter.

Revisit snacks

- ☐ Keep fresh fruits, portioned vegetables, homemade trail mix, or nuts and seeds handy to help crowd out sweet or savory snacks that have added sugar.

Consider salad dressings and sauces

- ☐ If you buy prepackaged salads, be sure to check the nutrition label for added sugar.
- ☐ Replace salad dressing with lower-sugar alternatives.
- ☐ Make a homemade weekly salad dressing from Chapter 17.
- ☐ Limit portion size of ketchup and barbecue sauce when dining out.

Evaluate your desserts

- ☐ Crowd out 1 dessert weekly with fresh or frozen fruit.
- ☐ Crowd out an additional dessert each week until you meet your AHA daily-added-sugar goals.
- ☐ Double-check portion size on sweets to be sure they fit into your AHA daily-added-sugar goals.

Review vitamins and vitamin drinks

☐ Review labels of any chewable, gummy, or powdered vitamins you take, looking for added sugar. If you find it, count it in your daily-added-sugar intake. Consider crowding out with a pill or capsule form of the vitamin that doesn't contain added sugar. If you are unable to swallow pills and don't want to continue consuming added sugar in your vitamins, contact your medical provider for other options.

Decrease sweeteners and sugar substitutes

☐ Week 1: Decrease sugar substitutes by one quarter each time you use them.

☐ Week 2: Decrease sugar by an additional quarter.

☐ Once you are consistently using half the synthetic sweetener you originally used, consider switching to a small amount of coconut sugar, honey, or maple syrup if you are medically able to do so. If you have a medical condition that affects the way you respond to sugar, consult your medical provider prior to switching sweeteners.

☐ Each week, decrease the amount of coconut sugar, honey, or maple syrup you are using until it fits well into your AHA daily-added-sugar goals.

Notes

[1] Magalie Lenoir, Fuschia Serre, Lauriane Cantin, and Serge H. Ahmed, "Intense sweetness surpasses cocaine reward," PLoS One 2, no. 8 (August 2007):e698, https://doi.org/10.1371/journal.pone.0000698.

[2] J. E. Beilharz, J. Maniam, and M. J. Morris, "Short-term exposure to a diet high in fat and sugar, or liquid sugar, selectively impairs hippocampal-dependent memory, with differential impacts on inflammation," Behav Brain Res 306 (2016):1–7, https://doi.org/10.1016/j.bbr.2016.03.018.

[3] Matthew P. Pase, Jayandra J. Himali, et al., "Sugary beverage intake and preclinical Alzheimer's disease in the community," Dement 13 (2017):955–964, https://doi.org/10.1016/j.jalz.2017.01.024.

CHAPTER 8

The Toxicity of Seed Oils

Seed oils, once heralded as healthy alternatives to traditional fats like butter and lard, strike at the core of brain health. Seed oils are extracted from vegetable seeds rather than from the grown and harvested vegetable itself. Common seed oils include canola (rapeseed) oil, corn oil, sesame oil, safflower oil, sunflower oil, rice bran oil, peanut oil, cottonseed oil, and soybean oil. Most "vegetable" oils on grocery store shelves are made of soybean oil. In contrast, olive oil and avocado oil are extracted from the flesh of the fruit rather than the seed, so they are not seed oils. The widespread adoption of seed oils as primary cooking oils and common ingredients in processed foods has inadvertently led to a nutritional imbalance that is detrimental to brain health. To understand seed oil's connection to the core processes of Alzheimer's disease, we need to know about omega fatty acids.

Understanding Unsaturated Fatty Acids

Omega-3 and omega-6 fats are **polyunsaturated fatty acids** (PUFAs), which play an essential role in various bodily functions. The body can't produce them on its own, so we need to get them from the foods we eat. Omega-3 PUFAs (think fish oils) are known for their anti-inflammatory properties as well as their role in supporting heart health and brain function. Omega-6 PUFAs are known for their ability to trigger inflammation in response to injury and support skin health and hormone production. For our discussion, it's important to remember that omega-3 PUFAs are anti-inflammatory while omega-6 PUFAs are pro-inflammatory. Historically, humans ingested omega PUFAs in a ratio of 2 (omega-6) to 1 (omega-3). That ratio reflects a healthy balance that keeps inflammation in check.

Seed oils are high in omega-6 PUFAs. Over the last century, our intake of seed oils has skyrocketed more than a thousandfold. Excessive consumption of pro-inflammatory omega-6 PUFAs without adequate anti-inflammatory omega-3s to balance them has dangerously shifted our omega-6-to-omega-3 intake ratio from 2 to 1 to a current ratio of 15 to 1! This skewed ratio fuels chronic inflammation in the body and brain.

Olive oil and avocado oil are different. They are composed mostly of a monounsaturated fatty acid (MUFA) called **oleic acid**, which is recognized for its wide variety of health benefits, including decreased risk of cognitive decline.[1] These non-seed oils also contain some omega-3 and omega-6 PUFAs. Overall, they are much lower in omega-6 PUFAs than seed oils are, and their ratio of omega-6 to omega-3 is optimally balanced to prevent inflammation.

Seed Oils: Production

The process of extracting oil from seeds requires high heat and chemical solvents. The solvents can strip away essential nutrients, while the high heat generates free radicals that cause oxidation. Refining these oils to be clear and odorless requires bleaching agents, which can leave traces of toxic residue behind.

Opting for extra-virgin olive oil or avocado oil helps you avoid these free radicals and toxins. Extracting oil from the flesh of these fruits requires less heat and chemical processing than seed oil extraction requires. As a result, these oils retain more of their naturally beneficial compounds, including antioxidants. We'll use these minimally processed oils to crowd out seed oils.

Seed Oils: Most Harmful When Heated

The predominant omega-6 PUFA in seed oils, **linoleic acid** (LA), poses the biggest dietary danger when it's heated. That's because LA is unstable at high temperatures and very susceptible to oxidation. When seed oils are heated, most of their LA becomes oxidized. One of the toxic free radicals kicked off by LA's oxidation reaction is a wickedly destructive compound called **4-hydroxynonenal** (HNE). Foods heated, sautéed, or fried in seed oils soak up dangerous HNE.

The digestive tract easily absorbs HNE from food. Once in the bloodstream, HNE travels throughout the body, setting off a firestorm of oxidation in every tissue it touches. As HNE circulates through arteries, it ricochets off the arterial walls, causing inflammation and initiating artery-clogging plaques. Upon reaching its final destination—the cells of every organ, including the brain, liver, heart, and kidneys—it harms proteins and DNA. Then it's stored in the cells and serves as an ongoing source of inflammation and oxidation. HNE is a truly vicious molecule that never misses an opportunity to cause harm.

Most restaurants—from fast-food to high-end—use seed oils in their fryers. Although it makes economic sense to reuse cooking oils for weeks, this repeated heating of cooking oils amplifies the amount of toxic HNE in them, which becomes concentrated in fried foods. By limiting or avoiding fried foods, you can lessen your exposure to HNE.

Seed Oils: Also a Threat When Not Heated

If you read ingredient labels on foods, you will find seed oils in most processed foods. The problem with unheated seed oils starts with the amount you are consuming. Like any fat you eat, if you consume more omega-6 PUFAs than you need, your body stores the extra fatty acids, including LA, in your fat cells.

The process of burning fats from storage to create energy is called ketosis. Ketosis is the only natural way to lose fat. Unfortunately, when LA goes through ketosis, the reaction is like when it's heated in a fryer: it generates HNE.

Your fat cells are like mini fryers in your body. When you eat salad dressings and processed foods that contain seed oils, LA gets stored in your fat cells—you're filling up your mini fryer vats with it. When your body fires up your metabolism and burns fat, that chemical reaction generates HNE. Even though your internal cell "fryers" don't heat up to 400 degrees like a restaurant fryer does, the HNE generated inside your body is just as destructive as the HNE you absorb from french fries and fried chicken.

Crowding out Seed Oil

Recognizing the role of seed oils in driving the core processes of Alzheimer's disease and reorienting your dietary patterns to restore proper omega fatty acid balance is crucial for nurturing cognitive vitality and well-being.

At Home

When you cook at home, you have more control over the oils you consume. Choose extra-virgin olive oil or avocado oil. These oils help you avoid imbalanced omega ratios and mitigate the inflammatory burden on the brain. Olive oil and avocado can both be used for salad dressings and low temperature cooking. However, for high temperature cooking, like roasting, sautéing, or air frying, avocado oil is the preferred choice due to its higher smoke point. (See page 64.)

Cutting down on the amount of seed oils you consume requires reading labels. So, it's time for another pantry and refrigerator audit. Set aside items you find with seed oils, then start crowding them out with each trip to the grocery store.

At the Grocery Store

Read labels and make conscious choices about what you put into your cart. As mentioned, seed oils are in nearly all processed foods. Shifting your diet to incorporate more whole, unprocessed foods will crowd out processed foods and lower your overall intake of seed oils.

Seed oils, like canola and safflower, are the dominant ingredient in most mayonnaise, salad dressings, and condiments. Thankfully, food manufacturers are starting to offer seed-oil-free options. Look for salad dressing and mayonnaise choices that are made with olive oil or avocado oil instead of canola oil. If you can't find salad dressings without seed oils, consider making your own dressing weekly. Added bonus: homemade dressings are usually more budget friendly than store-bought options.

When buying meat and dairy products, opt for those from grass-fed or pasture-raised animals when availability and affordability allow. Their meat and dairy products tend to have a healthier balance of omega-3 to omega-6 fatty acids than those from animals raised on grains.

When Dining Out

It's not always possible to avoid seed oils when dining out, but you can reduce your overall intake with a few simple strategies. Opting for grilled or steamed foods is an effective way to crowd out fried or sautéed foods that contain high levels of HNE.

Ask about the oils used to make salad dressings. In my experience, most restaurants' salad dressings and vinaigrettes use canola oil or a blend of olive oil and canola oil. You can cut down on seed oil intake by limiting portion size or asking for oil and vinegar (if they provide olive oil). If you are determined to aggressively cut seed oils after reading about how harmful they are, another option is to forgo dressing altogether and squeeze lemon wedges over your salad instead.

Final Word: Air Fryers

Cooking in an air fryer is a great way to minimize exposure to seed oils. Air fryers circulate hot air to cook food, producing a crispy outer layer similar to deep frying, but they use significantly less oil. Air frying requires just a few sprays or a teaspoon of oil to coat the food, compared to submerging food in a deep fryer full of oil and concentrated HNE.

When you use an air fryer, it's important to use an oil that has a smoke point above your cooking temperature. The smoke point is the temperature at which cooking oils start to break down, producing smoke, oxidants, and other harmful compounds. Avocado oil has a high smoke point (520°F) and is my preferred oil for high-heat cooking. Extra-virgin olive oil is not well-suited to air frying due to its relatively low smoke point (375°F).

Take Action: Tasks, Goals, and Mini Habits

Increase your intake of healthy oils, like olive oil and avocado oil, that are rich in oleic acid, have an optimally balanced ratio of omega-3 to omega-6 PUFAs, and reduce intake of seed oils that contain unhealthy levels of pro-inflammatory omega-6 PUFAs.

Perform a pantry and refrigerator/freezer audit

- ☐ Go through your cooking oils and set aside the seed oils: canola, corn, safflower, soybean, cottonseed, and vegetable oil. Replace with olive oil and avocado oil.

- ☐ Read labels on the other items in your refrigerator and pantry. Use a marker to circle the ingredient lists of foods that contain seed oils.

- ☐ When you finish an item with a circled ingredient list, take a picture of it with your phone.
- ☐ Add these pictures to the album you started in Chapter 7.
- ☐ Find seed-oil-free alternatives for as many of them as possible the next time you buy groceries.
- ☐ Miniaturize the task by addressing a different shelf or food category each day or each week. If you choose to go by categories, this list can guide you through pantry items:
  - o Crackers, chips, and nuts
  - o Cookies and candies
  - o Cereal, granola, granola bars, and protein bars
  - o Pasta sauce, salsa, and other sauces
  - o Peanut butter, other nut butters, and chocolate hazelnut spread
  - o Bread and tortillas
  - o Remaining items
- ☐ This list can guide you through refrigerator items:
  - o Salad dressings, marinades, sauces, and condiments
  - o Dairy, especially coffee creamers and processed cheese
  - o Breads and tortillas
  - o Remaining items

- ☐ This list can guide you through freezer items:
  - ○ Frozen meals and frozen pizza
  - ○ Frozen processed meats, such as breaded chicken and breakfast sausages
  - ○ Frozen desserts
  - ○ Remaining items

Crowd out seed oils when you cook

- ☐ Use extra-virgin olive oil for salad dressings, dips, and low-to-medium-heat cooking.
- ☐ Use avocado oil or refined olive oil for high-heat cooking, like sautéing and air frying.
- ☐ Opt to oven roast or air fry food instead of frying or sautéing.

Crowd out seed oils when you dine out

- ☐ Choose grilled or steamed foods instead of fried foods.
- ☐ If there is a fried food you love, like french fries or fried chicken, cutting it out altogether may not be reasonable. Decide how often you'll splurge and eat the item, then cut back gradually each week until you meet that goal.
- ☐ Ask about the oils used to make salad dressings and vinaigrettes. Opt for seed-oil-free options when available. Consider olive oil and vinegar or a squeeze of lemon juice on your salad if there are no other seed-oil-free choices.

Notes

[1] Keisuke Sakurai, Chutong Shen, Izumi Shiraishi, Noriko Inamura, and Tatsuhiro Hisatsune, "Consumption of Oleic Acid on the Preservation of Cognitive Functions in Japanese Elderly Individuals," Nutrients 13, no. 2 (January 2021):284, https://doi.org/10.3390/nu13020284.

CHAPTER 9

Time-Restricted Eating

When You Eat Is as Important as What You Eat

Fasting describes periods of time when you are not taking in calories, like when you are asleep at night. However, when we talk about fasting for health benefits, we are usually talking about more prolonged spans without food, typically beyond twelve hours. There are many different fasting patterns, but the Brain Health Action Plan focuses on one called time-restricted eating.

Time-restricted eating (TRE) is a fasting pattern that involves restricting your daily eating to a specific window of time, typically between eight and twelve hours. For example, if you choose a ten-hour window, you might eat all of your meals and snacks between nine a.m. and seven p.m., then fast for the fourteen hours between seven p.m. and nine a.m.

Fasting, and specifically TRE, are popular topics in magazines, on TV, and in social media. Are they just another diet fad or something you should consider?

To answer that question, we need to understand our ancestors.[1] Thousands of years ago, food was scarce. There was no farming, and food couldn't be preserved. Early humans roamed the Earth, hunting and gathering. They ate when food was available, which was when they killed a beast or came across some fruit. They often went for days without food. When they did eat, it was over the course of several hours. It was common for our distant ancestors to eat for four hours of a twenty-four-hour day. The other twenty hours were spent fasting.

Our food supply has evolved more quickly than we have. Most of our genes are the same as they were thousands of years ago, when food was scarce, while many people now live in food abundance. With the constant availability of food, we might be eating for sixteen or eighteen hours of a twenty-four-hour period. Although we spend most of our day eating, our genes are still geared for spending the majority of our day fasting.

This mismatch between our genes and our modern food supply contributes to chronic diseases like diabetes, heart disease, and Alzheimer's disease.

Fasting to treat disease goes back to the ancient Greek physician Hippocrates. He treated patients with fasting to reduce fevers in 400 BC. Since the early 1900s, physicians have used a version of fasting in some epilepsy patients to reduce seizures.[2]

Fueling the Brain

There are only two molecules that can fuel the brain: glucose (sugar from carbohydrates) and ketones (from fats). If both are present in your bloodstream after a meal, your default setting is to use glucose as your primary energy source. You use ketones as your primary fuel only when no glucose is available. **Ketosis** is the term for the metabolic state when your body and brain use stored fats as your primary energy source. That's when you reap the health benefits of fasting. How you switch fuels throughout the day is a complex process that's worth understanding.

> *The keto diet is based on the principles of fasting. It's a high-fat, low-carbohydrate eating plan that starves the body of glucose to force it to use ketones for energy. While some aspects of this diet support brain health, the severe carbohydrate restriction can lead to nutritional deficiencies that impair brain function.*

As you eat throughout the day, you take in a broad array of nutrients and power your body with glucose from carbohydrates. After you stop eating, it takes a while for your body to switch to using ketones and get the brain health benefits. The carbohydrate calories from your last meal of the day give you energy for a couple of hours. Once those are used up, your body starts using sugar that was stored in your liver during the daytime. The sugar in your liver is stored for this purpose and is called glycogen. Typically, there is enough liver glycogen to maintain blood glucose levels and power your system for ten to fourteen hours. Since glycogen is converted to glucose for energy, your body is still generating insulin to move glucose into cells. When the supply of glycogen in the liver is depleted, your body makes an important metabolic shift to ketosis. With no sugar in your bloodstream and no glycogen left in your liver, your body turns to your fat cells for energy. Fat cells release stored fatty acids into the bloodstream, which are converted to ketones in the liver. Your body remains in ketosis, using ketones for energy, as long as no glucose is available. When you have breakfast—literally, break your fast—with carbohydrates, your body and brain immediately switch back to using glucose as fuel and stop using ketones.

The Brain Benefits of Time-Restricted Eating

Restoring Insulin Sensitivity

Consistently high sugar intake in the modern American diet leads to chronically high insulin levels. High levels of insulin overstimulate the cells to try to take in sugar, which causes stress at the cellular level. Stressed cells become less responsive to insulin's signals over time, leaving sugar in the bloodstream that should have been ushered into cells by insulin. High blood sugar that isn't getting into cells triggers the body to produce even more insulin, and the cycle goes on. Eventually, your body can become insulin resistant from constant exposure to sugar and insulin, and that can start you on the path toward type 2 diabetes.

Time-restricted eating can get you into ketosis and give your body a break from sugar and insulin. This alleviates stress on your cells so they can reset and restore their responsiveness to insulin.

> *Alzheimer's disease has sometimes been referred to as "type 3 diabetes" because high-sugar diets can cause neurons to become insulin resistant. The most important brain benefit of time-restricted eating is restoring the brain's natural insulin response.*

Cellular Cleaning and Repair

Fasting doesn't just help burn fat and restore insulin sensitivity; it also activates a cleaning system in the body that removes damaged proteins from cells. This is important because the buildup of damaged proteins—beta-amyloid and tau among them—can accelerate brain disease and aging. Researchers have found that fasting can also improve diabetes, heart disease, hypertension, and cholesterol.[3]

Consultation

It's crucial to consider your individual needs and medical history prior to adopting these practices. Consult your healthcare provider prior to starting any TRE regimen.

Separating the Last Calories from the First Calories

Let's say you finish dinner at eight p.m. and don't have any more calories before bedtime. Your body would run on stored liver sugar until sometime between five a.m. and nine a.m. the following day. If you eat breakfast at seven a.m., you may not have burned through the supply of liver glycogen. That means your body doesn't get a break from glucose and has no chance to burn fat or restore its sensitivity to insulin.

As mentioned, most of us eat for the majority of a twenty-four-hour period. The first step to giving your body a break from running on sugar is to even up the eating and fasting windows. Separate the last calories of the night from the first calories of the morning by twelve hours. This pattern is referred to as 12:12 (twelve hours eating and twelve hours not eating). You may have just burned through the liver glycogen during that twelve-hour period.

After practicing this for a period of time, and if your health care provider has cleared you to incorporate a longer fasting period, you can try to stretch the fasting period another hour or two. Many people find that 14:10 (fourteen hours between last nighttime calories and first calories of the morning and ten hours eating) is achievable. Once accustomed to this TRE pattern, some people find it beneficial to stretch to a 15:9 or even 16:8 pattern one day per week, again under medical supervision.

Speaking personally, of all the interventions in this book, I noticed the biggest improvement in my mental focus and body composition when I adopted TRE. A secondary benefit of following my TRE schedule is that I realized how many empty calories I had been consuming after dinner. Eating dessert, snacking as I made my kids lunches, or having a glass of wine after dinner added calories to my system at the end of the day, when I need that fuel the least.

If TRE isn't appropriate for you—due to either medical concerns or personal preferences—your brain can still benefit from the concepts discussed in this chapter. Consider your evenings and your mornings. A couple of small tweaks can bring brain health benefits. In the evening, be mindful to not snack after dinner. Swap high-sugar beverages or alcohol for mineral water or decaffeinated tea. In the morning, you can make small but beneficial changes even if you eat breakfast less than twelve hours after you finished eating the night before. Ease your system back into glucose metabolism by eating a high-protein breakfast instead of jarring your system into glucose overdrive with a sugary or high-carbohydrate breakfast.

Don't Eat in Your Fasting Window, and Don't Fast in Your Eating Window

Once you set your TRE schedule, do your best to stick to it most days. Keep in mind that your fasting window doesn't start until you stop eating at the end of the day. Having a late-night snack or a drink with calories pushes your last calories of the day later. If you're trying to maintain your fasting window, then the time you start eating the next morning will be delayed, which can make for a rough morning.

Similarly, once you break your fast in the morning, you are in your eating window. During your eating window, you should be taking in all the nutrition your brain and body need. If you embrace a TRE schedule, there will be days when you break your fast earlier than you would like to. Accept the change in your schedule and go about your day as usual. Don't skip meals during your eating window to try to make up for the early breakfast. Not only will you be missing the opportunity to eat valuable nutrients, but you also won't get back to ketosis during that time, and you'll likely feel hungry and deprived.

Take Action: Tasks, Goals, and Mini Habits

With the guidance of your health care provider, determine the level of time-restricted fasting, if any, that is appropriate for you

- ☐ Contact your health care provider to discuss time-restricted eating.
- ☐ Follow your provider's advice in setting your TRE schedule, gradually working up to the level they recommend using the suggested steps below.

With the guidance of your health care provider, incorporate the level of time-restricted fasting that is appropriate for you

- ☐ Circle the pattern you have been cleared for and cross out the schedules below that exceed it.
- ☐ If medically cleared for 12:12 TRE pattern:
    - o Set your 12:12 schedule. There are two ways to approach this. You can choose the 12 hours of the day in which you will consume all of your calories (time-based option). If you need more flexibility, you can focus on separating your last calories of the night from your first calories of the day by 12 hours (flexible time option). Note the time you finish calories at the end of the day to

determine what time you will break your fast the following morning. During your fasting window, you can have water, tea, or black coffee (decaffeinated in the evening!)—anything without calories.

☐ If medically cleared for 14:10 TRE pattern:

   o After you have been following 12:12 TRE pattern for two to four weeks, set your 14:10 schedule. Utilize the same option that worked best for you when setting your 12:12 schedule, either time-based or flexible, to set your 14:10 TRE pattern.

☐ If medically cleared for 15:9 or 16:8 one day per week:

   o Once you are accustomed to 14:10 TRE, you may find that you aren't hungry when your eating window is scheduled to start. If you feel well, you have the option to postpone breakfast by an hour or two. This is an optional fasting threshold that may be unrealistic for most people.

If your medical provider determines that time-restricted eating is not appropriate for you:

☐ In the evening, reduce snacks and drinks between the end of dinner and bedtime. Use water, mineral water, decaffeinated tea or coffee,

☐ or decaffeinated black coffee to crowd out drinks that have calories.

☐ In the morning, start off the day with a savory, high-protein breakfast instead of a high-carbohydrate or sugary breakfast.

NOTES

[1] Matthew C. L. Phillips, "Fasting as a Therapy in Neurological Disease," Nutrients 11, no. 10 (October 2019):2501, https://doi.org/10.3390/nu11102501.
[2] Adam L. Hartman and Eileen P. G. Vining, "Clinical Aspects of the Ketogenic Diet," Epilepsia 48 (2007):31–42, https://doi.org/10.1111/j.1528-1167.2007.00914.x.
[3] Rafael de Cabo and Mark P. Mattson, "Effects of Intermittent Fasting on Health, Aging, and Disease," N Engl J Med. 381, no. 26 (December 2019):2541–2551, https://doi.org/10.1056/nejmra1905136.

CHAPTER 10

Prepare for Success

Breaking up with the Convenience Lifestyle

Breakups are difficult, and habits are hard to break—especially when the habits are easy and confront you everywhere you go. Leaving the convenience lifestyle can make you feel like you are heading to an inconvenient lifestyle. The good news is that eating healthy doesn't have to be cumbersome. A few simple strategies can help ease the burden of optimizing your nutrition.

Preparation Is Key

Eating brain-healthy meals and snacks requires a return to whole, unprocessed foods. By definition, these aren't the grab-and-go options that you can pick up last minute from the vending machine at work. **Meal planning, utilizing leftovers,** and **preparing fresh fruits and vegetables** play a pivotal role in helping you embrace better food choices and avoid processed foods. Spending a few minutes during your week to plan and prep will ease the burden of making healthier choices.

Meal Planning

Not only is meal planning a huge time-saver, it promotes healthier eating habits throughout the week in several ways. When you plan your week of meals and snacks, you are more likely to create balanced dishes with nutritious ingredients and appropriate portion sizes. Knowing what you are going to eat makes you less likely to make impulsive, unhealthy choices that often happen when you're hungry and unprepared. Meal planning reduces the expense and stress that is caused by last-minute decisions about what to eat. Another benefit is that planning ahead helps reduce food waste.

It's just as important to **plan your snacks** for the week. Consider your cravings throughout the day. Plan snacks that will meet those cravings and provide nutritious benefits. Plan fresh fruit snacks, yogurt, or chia parfaits for the time of day when you tend to crave sweets. Hummus and veggies, air-popped popcorn, whole-grain seed-oil-free crackers, nuts, and homemade trail mix are great snacks to satisfy savory, salty, or crunchy cravings. See the recipe section for suggestions.

Set aside time to meal plan before you go to the grocery store. Fortunately, meal planning doesn't have to take all day, and you don't have to start from scratch. Online meal planners are a great time-saving hack. You can select your nutrition preferences, anything from omnivore to vegetarian to paleo, and your desired level of cooking complexity. Meal-planning websites will generate a weekly meal plan, including recipes and a shopping list. Some will even link to your favorite grocery store and add the items to your cart for online shopping and pickup.

Cook Once, Eat Twice

Eating better typically involves cooking more meals at home. As you meal plan for the week, maximize the return on your efforts by cooking large dinners so you'll have leftovers on hand for healthy, low-effort lunches. Prepare your lunch for the next day as you are cleaning up dinner. My favorite strategy is "saladizing" my dinner for lunch the next day. I fill an airtight container with a couple of handfuls of pre-washed lettuce, some veggies from dinner, and a bit of the leftovers from the protein I had with dinner. In the morning, I add a splash of seed-oil-free dressing before I leave for work.

Prepping Fresh Fruits and Vegetables

Prepping fresh fruits and vegetables right after returning from the grocery store can be a game-changer for eating healthier and saving time throughout the week. Eating healthy meals relies more heavily on preparing foods at home rather than buying prepared foods. Cooking takes time and effort, especially if all the prep work is done at each meal. The key to success in cooking meals from whole foods is to prepare components ahead of time. When you return home from grocery shopping, set aside some time to prep some of the fruits and vegetables you purchased. Washing and cutting the week's vegetables at one time and storing them in the refrigerator takes less time than preparing the vegetables you need for one meal at the time you are cooking. It's sometimes hard to get motivated to do the prep work up front, but that time invested at the beginning of the week saves so much time throughout the week. It's truly a stitch in time that saves nine.

When you are done washing and cutting fruits and veggies, it's a great time to make some snacks for the week. Portioning fruits and veggies into grab-and-go containers or resealable bags makes them convenient for healthy snacking, whether at home, at work, or on the go.

Evening Routine

Set aside a few minutes in the evening to review your meal plan for the next day. Be sure that your snacks and lunch are ready for the next day and that you have the ingredients you need for the next night's dinner. This helps prevent morning stress and reduces the likelihood of making unhealthy last-minute choices the following day.

Take Action: Tasks, Goals, and Mini Habits

Prepare to prepare

- ☐ Evaluate your storage containers to determine if you have enough to store the fruits and vegetables for the week's meals. If you're at that point where you have a million lids and no containers, treat yourself to an updated set. Consider glass or BPA-free plastic.

☐ Check out online meal-planning websites.

Prep for the week

☐ Week 1: Set aside a half hour after returning from the grocery store to prep fruits and vegetables for the week's meals.

☐ Week 2: Plan and purchase midmorning snacks for the week, like fresh fruit. Do any prep that is needed when you return from the grocery store, and portion them into resealable bags so they are ready to grab and take with you.

☐ Week 3: Plan and purchase afternoon snacks for the week. Prepare, portion, and package them as you did with midmorning snacks. Consider veggies, nuts, crackers, beef jerky, or deli meat and cheese roll-ups.

☐ Week 4: Make a homemade salad dressing* for the week.

☐ Week 5: If you're trying to crowd out sugary desserts with fruit, prep those fruits along with those for snacks and other meals.

☐ Week 6: Prepare a make-ahead breakfast, like chia pudding,* to crowd out flavored yogurt, or choose baked oatmeal* to crowd out sugary cereal. Either of these will keep in the refrigerator for several days.

*See Chapter 17 for recipes.

CHAPTER 11

Optimal Sleep

"Addressing other putative risk factors for dementia, like sleep, through lifestyle interventions, will improve general health."
—The Lancet Commission

Even just one night of bad sleep changes the way your brain works. When you wake up in an unrefreshed fog, that is a day you'll avoid tasks that demand brainpower, like working on taxes. You are more likely to put those chores off and hope you'll sleep better the next night. That's the short-term impact of poor sleep. When you have night after night of poor sleep, however, there are serious long-term consequences.

Sleep: The Basics

Getting enough sleep—both duration and quality—allows you to wake up feeling refreshed and promotes brain health.

Duration

The general recommendation for optimal brain health is to aim for seven to nine hours of sleep nightly. Within that range, finding the right amount of sleep that leaves you refreshed, alert, and productive the next day will vary based on your individual needs, medical considerations, and lifestyle factors.

Quality

Quality of sleep refers to how effectively you move through the different sleep stages and how long you spend in each one.

Sleep Stages

The four stages of sleep are unimaginatively named stages 1, 2, 3, and rapid eye movement (REM) sleep. Each stage is unique and contributes special benefits in terms of memory, brain health, and how refreshed and restored you feel in the morning. Here's what happens in your brain during these stages.

Stage 1: This is the couple of minutes of drowsiness on the way to falling asleep. Your body temperature starts to drop, and your breathing becomes more regular. Muscles start to relax and might twitch. Not much happens in the brain. In fact, you might not even feel like you're asleep during this stage. Approximately thirty minutes to an hour (5% to 10% of your sleep) is spent in stage 1.

Stage 2: This stage, called light sleep, consumes half of your night. Your body temperature drops a bit more, and your heart rate slows. Your brain processes information you learned in the day to form memories. About 50%, or around four hours of your sleep, is stage 2.

Stage 3: This is deep sleep. Your brain continues to work on storing memories and undergoes a unique and important deep cleaning. Deep sleep actually causes some of the supporting cells of the brain to temporarily shrink. This creates more space between the neurons. Cerebrospinal fluid (CSF) flows into these spaces, bathing the neurons in clean CSF and removing metabolic waste and toxins, including beta-amyloid, that accumulate in the neurons during the day.[1] This cleaning mechanism helps the neurons reset themselves for the next day and is separate from the cellular cleaning-and-repair process that is activated by fasting. Although sleep needs can vary from person to person, getting one to two hours of stage 3 sleep is enough for most people to wake up feeling refreshed the next morning. We get most of our stage 3 deep sleep in the first half of the night. The good news for people whose sleep pattern includes waking up around two a.m. or three a.m. is that they have likely gotten most of the deep sleep they need by then. About 20%, or one to two hours, of sleep is spent in deep sleep.

Rapid eye movement (REM) sleep: REM is when you dream. The brain is very active during REM sleep—as active as it is when you are awake. Although your eyes move a lot during this stage, your body is temporarily paralyzed. When you want to run or shout in a dream but can't, you are feeling the paralysis of your body during REM sleep.

In REM sleep, your brain continues to form memories, but those memories are more likely to be emotional. We typically reach the first REM stage about ninety minutes after falling asleep. That stage is usually short. REM cycles and dreams get longer in the second half of the night. About 25%, or close to two hours, of sleep is spent in REM.

Mapping Sleep

A hypnogram is a graphic representation of sleep. By monitoring brain activity, muscle movement, heart rate, and breathing rate, we can map out how long someone slept and record how much time they spent in each sleep stage. As you look at the normal hypnogram below, you'll notice the characteristic shapes that are formed as we transition in and out of different sleep stages. Seeing the pattern that looks like upside-down skyscrapers makes it easy to understand why doctors refer to sleep patterns, including depth and length of sleep, as "sleep architecture." The diagram below is an example of a normal hypnogram.

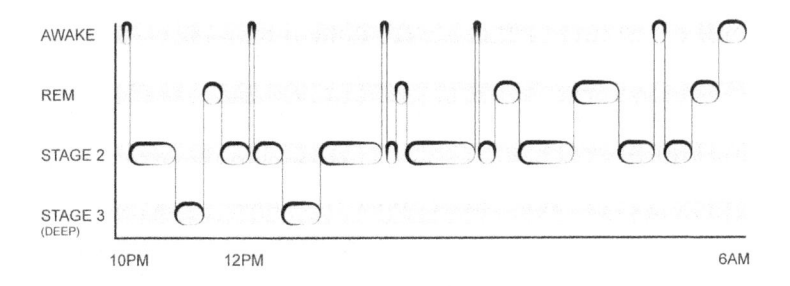

The hypnogram above shows that this person slept over seven hours and moved efficiently through the various sleep stages. They spent about half the night in stage 2 sleep, and the other half was split between REM and stage 3. A person with this sleep pattern would wake up feeling well-rested and restored.

This is an abnormal hypnogram:

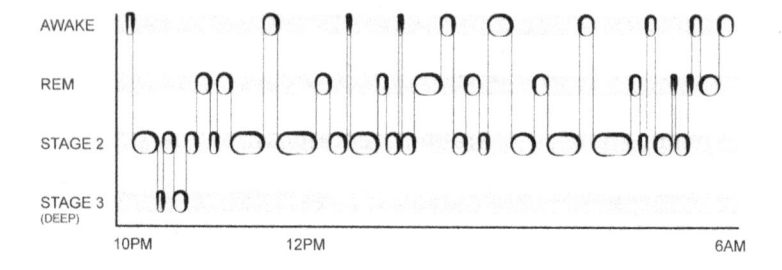

The hypnogram above reveals numerous small awakenings throughout the night that prevented adequate deep sleep and REM sleep. Many things that interrupt sleep can cause this pattern; this one is the result of sleeping in a room that was too hot. A person with this sleep map would likely wake up feeling tired and unrefreshed.

You might be wondering what your sleep cycles look like. In the past, hypnograms were done only in sleep centers. Now, advances in personal technology allow us to gather our own sleep data. An entire industry of wearable health-tracking devices has emerged. These include smartwatches, fitness bands, and rings, most of which track daytime activity as well as sleep patterns. An up-to-date list of some of these devices is available on my website: www.brainhealthactionplan.com/smarttech

Circadian Rhythm

Environmental cues tell your brain when it should be awake or asleep. Two hormones translate environmental cues into sleep and wake cycles: cortisol and melatonin. They shift throughout the twenty-four-hour day to establish your circadian rhythm. Cortisol dominates the daytime, and melatonin dominates the nighttime.

Cortisol tells the brain to be active. High cortisol levels are associated with wakefulness, stress, and action. Low cortisol levels are associated with relaxation and sleep. Cortisol rises in the morning to help you wake up. It decreases throughout the day. It is lowest in the evening, which signals your brain to relax and go to sleep.

Melatonin tells your brain when it's dark. In low light, the pineal gland (located right behind your eyes) produces melatonin, which makes you sleepy. When it's light, your eyes prevent the pineal gland from producing melatonin so your brain doesn't get a sleepiness signal in the daytime.

This schematic shows what the levels of cortisol and melatonin should look like over a twenty-four-hour period:

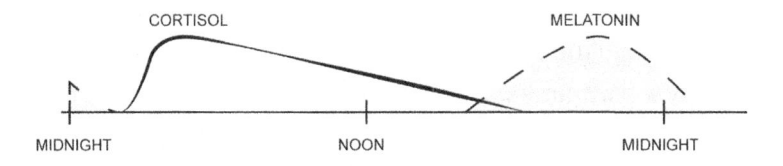

Our modern lifestyle is upsetting the balance of cortisol and melatonin. If you're stressed all day long and working on your computer into the evenings, your levels will look more like this:

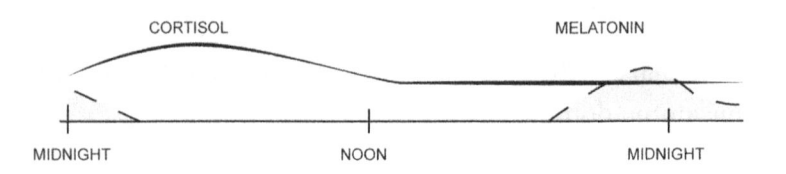

```
           CORTISOL                    MELATONIN
    MIDNIGHT          NOON             MIDNIGHT
```

Cortisol Shouldn't Be High at Night

Stress makes your cortisol levels high. We were designed to have infrequent, quick spikes of cortisol in response to threats, like wild animals. Our modern lifestyle is filled with constant moderate stress, which keeps cortisol high throughout the day and into the evening. High cortisol levels at night make it hard for you to get to sleep and stay asleep.

Melatonin Shouldn't Be Low at Night

Your brain was designed to produce high levels of melatonin at night to make you sleepy. However, in our modern world, electronics brighten the evening environment and prevent the pineal gland from producing melatonin. Once you turn off TVs, computers, and smartphones for the day, it takes some time for melatonin to build up. Evening screen time not only delays your melatonin peak, but it also causes the peak to be lower than it would have been without all the direct light stimulation after dusk.

Midlife Sleep Challenges

Many of us notice a change in how well we sleep as we move into midlife. Overall, older adults tend to sleep less, and their sleep is characterized by more awakenings during the night. There are several main contributors to this unfortunate phenomenon. The hormonal changes caused by perimenopause and menopause in women and by andropause in men can disrupt sleep. Health issues, like chronic back pain and arthritis, can make it hard to find a comfortable sleeping position or can awaken us with discomfort in the middle of the night. For many, midlife is characterized by increased responsibilities, like managing career demands while simultaneously raising children and caring for aging parents. Heightened midlife stress can upset the cortisol balance and impair sleep.

Foster Healthy Sleep Habits

Creating a proper sleep environment for yourself is called **sleep hygiene**. Your brain is taking cues from the environment that should be setting the stage for relaxed sleep. In midlife, you may need to take a more active approach to creating cues that signal the brain to go to sleep. These are the steps you can take to improve your sleep:

Create an Evening Wind-Down Routine

Set a good routine full of sleep cues in the evening. Start with a consistent bedtime. Based on that, set a time to stop taking in calories (ideally three hours before bedtime). During those three hours, you can drink water or have decaffeinated tea but nothing with calories. Then set a time to stop looking at TV, computer, and smartphone screens (ideally one to two hours before bedtime). That allows your melatonin to start rising naturally.

In that two-hour quiet period between screen time and bedtime, you can add more sleeping cues: read a book, enjoy decaffeinated tea, take a warm bath, meditate, or pray. All are good ways to prepare your brain and body for a good night's sleep.

Relax Your Mind

Breath work, meditation, and prayer help alleviate insomnia.

Breath work, or intentional breathing, deactivates your fight-or-flight sympathetic nervous system and turns on your rest-and-digest parasympathetic nervous system. Two easy patterns that bring about relaxation are box breathing and 4-7-8 relaxation breathing.

Box breathing: Inhale for four seconds, hold for four seconds, exhale for four seconds, hold for four seconds. Start with ten rounds and work up to ten minutes as you become more comfortable.

4-7-8 relaxation breathing: Inhale for four seconds, hold for seven seconds, exhale for eight seconds. As with box breathing, start with ten rounds and work up to ten minutes as you become more comfortable.

Try these when you go to bed to see which helps you get to sleep faster. They are also helpful when you are trying to fall back asleep in the middle of the night.

Meditating and praying are other ways to help your mind disconnect from the busy thoughts of the day and let go of worry. If meditation and prayer are not already part of your lifestyle, understand that it will take practice and consistency to see results. Use an online guided meditation to help you get to sleep. Once you are proficient at the practice, meditate on your own to drift off to sleep so you don't have to keep electronics by your bedside. You can also meditate to fall back asleep after an awakening or a trip to the restroom. It may be impractical to use guided meditation in the middle of the night because you might wake your bed partner. Instead, train yourself to meditate during the day or evening so that when you need to meditate in the middle of the night to get back to sleep, you know what to do. Having a simple go-to meditation will settle your mind and can be extremely helpful for attaining restorative sleep.

Avoid Late-Night Snacks and Nightcaps

It's counterproductive to rev up your metabolism with calories late in the evening. Snack calories consumed during that time tend to be empty and unnecessary anyway. Eating prior to bedtime stimulates your body and doesn't promote true relaxation. Similarly, alcohol may feel relaxing, but it can lessen REM sleep and lead to insomnia.[2] As noted previously, I recommend not consuming calories for two to three hours before going to bed. Set your dinnertime based on your bedtime so that your meal concludes at least two hours prior to bedtime.

Curate an Ideal Sleep Environment

Make it dark: Your bedroom should be dark. You awaken several times during the night between sleep cycles, whether you realize it or not. Early in life, you awaken, briefly open your eyes, and go back to sleep without even registering the fact that you awoke. By midlife, people often become aware of awakening and may have trouble getting back to sleep. To prevent awareness of awakening, make your bedroom as dark as possible. When you first go to bed, the bedroom seems dark compared to how light it was before you turned off the lights. However, in the middle of the night, your room may be lighter than you realized. The small lights on smoke detectors, clocks, and TVs can emit significant light in your bedroom. You can dim clocks and cover any sensor lights on TVs with black electrical tape. It is not advised, however, to cover up lights on safety equipment, such as smoke detectors or carbon monoxide detectors.

Wearing a sleep mask is another option for blocking your brain from registering brief wakefulness between sleep cycles. Contoured sleep masks are elevated over the eyes, which lets you open your eyes at night without seeing any light. If this helps you get through just one of the awakenings without becoming wide awake, that makes a difference.

Make it quiet: Take steps to minimize ambient noise that may be bothering you at night. Keep cell phones out of your bedroom, and turn off electronics while sleeping. Noise from outside your house may be notable and difficult to control. If there is outside noise that affects your bedroom, consider masking it with white noise or pink noise.

White noise makers are widely available and provide more consistent sounds to combat variable environment sounds. White noise makers have been shown to improve sleep quality. Pink noise makers are newer on the scene. Their sound frequencies promote stable deep sleep and are more relaxing than those of white noise. Look for videos of white noise and pink noise online and listen to them on a phone to determine which works better for you. Then, I recommend buying a machine that produces your preferred tones so you can again remove your phone from your bedroom.

Wearing earplugs is not a great idea because they might prevent you from hearing important emergency sounds, such as a smoke detector or house alarm system.

Train your brain to stop thinking in bed: Do you wake up at night with an active mind, solving problems at two a.m.? You are not alone! Working, playing computer games, Web browsing, and watching TV in bed can inadvertently train your brain to stay active and alert when you hit the pillow. Restore the connection between going to bed and relaxing or disconnecting from purposeful thinking. The first step is to remove electronics from the bedroom. If you read, work, watch television, or surf the Web in the evening, do that in another room before you start your bedtime wind-down routine.

Consistency Is Key

Follow a consistent sleep schedule. Just as you set a time to wake up, set a bedtime based on a goal of sleeping seven to eight hours nightly. If you keep to this schedule most nights, it will help retrain your body to follow its natural circadian rhythms.

Work on Your Circadian Rhythm in the Daytime

Fostering a healthy circadian rhythm in the daytime can also help you sleep better at night. Set aside ten to fifteen minutes within the first three hours of your morning to get exposure to sunlight. If you live in a climate where this is hard to do in the winter months, a light box can be a helpful tool.

Sleep Aids

If you are still having trouble getting to sleep or staying asleep even after optimizing sleep hygiene, it may be time to consider taking a sleep aid. All supplements and over-the-counter medications carry the risk of side effects and drug interactions and must be discussed with your physician prior to starting. The following is information about why your physician might suggest one of the following but should not be taken as medical advice. Always consult your medical provider before starting supplements or over-the-counter medications.

Let's Revisit Melatonin

Doctors sometimes recommend melatonin to reestablish a healthy circadian rhythm. In adulthood, the amount of melatonin produced by the pineal gland is about 0.3 milligrams. Most melatonin supplements range from 1 to 10 milligrams. This is quite a bit higher than the amount of melatonin we produce. Melatonin beyond what is needed for sleep can result in other positive effects on the body and brain. Scientists continue to discover beneficial effects, including melatonin's antiviral and antiaging actions.

Recent animal studies in mice likely to develop Alzheimer's disease showed that melatonin helps clear beta-amyloid and tau from the brain during deep sleep.[3] Studies on humans to determine the optimal dosing to fight neurodegenerative diseases are underway.

Magnesium

Magnesium relaxes the body and mind. Not only does it aid with melatonin production, but it also works through the neurotransmitter GABA to calm the nervous system. Studies show that magnesium decreases nighttime awakenings and helps people sleep deeper and longer.[4]

L-theanine

L-theanine is an amino acid discussed in Chapter 6 that is primarily found in tea. If you drink decaffeinated tea in the evening, you're probably already experiencing the relaxation-promoting benefits of L-theanine.

L-theanine improves sleep quality and helps us fall asleep faster through several mechanisms. It decreases the stress hormone cortisol, which can interfere with sleep. Like magnesium, L-theanine also increases GABA to calm the nervous system.

Ashwagandha

Ashwagandha is an herb used in Ayurvedic medicine. Like L-theanine, ashwagandha reduces cortisol and promotes GABA to calm the mind and promote sleep. Some people also notice decreased feelings of anxiety while taking ashwagandha.

Valerian Root

Valerian root helps some people fall asleep faster. Studies show that it improves sleep quality by increasing GABA.

Over-the-Counter Sleep Meds and "P.M." Pain Meds

Many people take over-the-counter (OTC) sleep medications to help them get their zzz's or OTC pain medications that have the "P.M." tag added to them because they cause drowsiness. These medications usually contain either diphenhydramine or doxylamine, which are antihistamines that cause drowsiness. These are called first-generation antihistamines because they have been around since the mid-1900s. They were originally intended to treat allergies. However, they easily cross the BBB and interact with receptors in the brain,[5] resulting in the side effect of sedation. Drug companies and doctors harnessed that side effect to help people get to sleep. Although they are widely available and relatively effective, they have additional side effects that upset the neurotransmitter balance in the brain. Medications that block histamines in the brain also block compounds in the choline family. That has ramifications for brain function because one of the most important cholines is acetylcholine—a neurotransmitter in the brain involved in memory. In fact, prolonging the effect of acetylcholine is how many of the Alzheimer's medications work. Although sleep is important for brain health, you must balance your need for sleep with your need for healthy neurotransmitter balance. Focusing your efforts on optimizing sleep hygiene and considering natural approaches to triggering drowsiness is a better way to promote sleep without directly hampering neuron function in the brain. (Nonsedating antihistamines do not disrupt cholines and are discussed in Chapter 14.)

Reversing Brain Fog

I have witnessed the profound effect these medications can have on cognitive function. I've had several patients referred to me for dementia who were taking OTC sleep aids, certain allergy medications, or one of the "P.M." pain relievers to sleep. In each case, once we stopped the medication, these patients returned to normal.

You might be wondering how they and their partner failed to recognize that the medicine was causing cognitive impairment. Brain dysfunction from these medications can sneak up on people because the speed of clearing medications from the system slows with age. Younger people have more rapid detoxification systems in the liver. If they take diphenhydramine at night, they usually clear it from their blood by the morning. However, as people age and their medication detox processes become more sluggish, they are more likely to wake up in the morning with diphenhydramine still circulating in their blood. Then, the next evening, they layer on more sleep medicine, and it builds up. Hence, an OTC medicine that someone has taken for a decade can cause a new side effect. Most drugs are tested on young or middle-aged folks. As a result, too little data exists on how medications affect seniors. Experience has taught us that just because someone has tolerated a medication well in the past, we cannot assume they will continue to have no side effects from it as they age.

Sedatives

Zolpidem, diazepam, and alprazolam are prescribed widely in the US to treat anxiety and insomnia. They modulate neurotransmitters, decreasing communication between neurons in the brain. These medications are sedative hypnotics, meaning they are calming and make us sleep. Unfortunately, the sleep they induce does not have the usual pattern of sleep we've discussed. Some people use these in small doses to block anxiety that prevents them from falling asleep. Then, at some point in the night, the medicine washes out of their body, and sleep normalizes. Unfortunately, these medications can interfere with the deep brain-cleansing sleep in the first half of the night. Although the long-term effects of taking these medications are controversial in terms of risk of dementia, the short-term side effects include confusion. It is important to consult your provider to find suitable medications for your particular health situation.

If you take one of these, consider incorporating the sleep hygiene recommendations, and work closely with your provider to minimize medications and find the best fit for you.

Final Word: Sleep Disorders

Sleep disorders often go unrecognized. They can cause memory impairment in the short term and increase the risk of Alzheimer's disease in the long term. Although most people will never experience a sleep disorder, they are worth mentioning, as diagnosis and treatment can be life changing.

REM Sleep Disorder

When you dream in REM sleep, you are paralyzed. Your brain stem blocks your brain from commanding your body to move or speak. We have all had the experience while dreaming that we needed to run or yell but couldn't. That sensation is due to brain stem blocking. If this brain stem blocking mechanism isn't working properly, you can talk, yell, and flail wildly as you dream. People have thrown themselves out of bed or punched their spouse while dreaming due to this problem. If you or your bed partner acts out or yells out dreams frequently, it's important to discuss it with your health provider.

Sleep Apnea

Apneic spells are periods during sleep when breathing pauses. They may be silent or accompanied by choking sounds. Apneic spells can be frightening for a bed partner who is waiting for their loved one to start breathing again. They can also be a symptom of underlying sleep apnea. Snoring is another symptom of sleep apnea. However, not all snoring equates to sleep apnea. The best way to figure out if snoring is due to a sleep disorder is to have a sleep evaluation.

Sleep apnea interrupts sleep cycles, preventing people from attaining deep sleep and its restorative benefits. Untreated sleep apnea is associated with increased buildup of beta-amyloid and an increased risk of Alzheimer's disease.[6] Treating sleep apnea can help restore healthy sleep cycles and reduce the risk of Alzheimer's disease.[7]

Take Action: Tasks, Goals, and Mini Habits

Assess your sleep

- ☐ If you have a bed partner, ask them if you snore, choke, skip breaths, or act out your dreams. If you do, make an appointment to discuss these with your healthcare provider.

Optimize sleep hygiene

Set your schedule

- ☐ Set your bedtime: _____
- ☐ Set the time you will wake up. Aim for 7 to 9 hours of sleep: _____
- ☐ Set your dinnertime 2 to 3 hours before bedtime: _____
- ☐ Set the time you will turn off electronics (ideally 1 to 2 hours before bedtime): _____

Create your wind-down routine 1 to 2 hours before bedtime

- ☐ Determine what you will drink during your wind-down time: water, decaffeinated tea or coffee, mineral water (beverages with no caffeine and no calories).
- ☐ Determine your relaxing wind-down activities: reading, taking a bath, etc.

Curate your sleep environment

- ☐ Darken your room. Dim clocks, and turn off or put electrical tape over any lights on your TV or other electronics.
- ☐ Order a sleep mask. It may take a week to get used to wearing it and see the sleep benefits.
- ☐ Make your room quiet; remove electronics.
- ☐ If your room is still noisy, try pink or white noise on your phone.
- ☐ If possible, order whichever type of noise maker you prefer so you can remove your phone from your room.

Retrain your brain

- ☐ Keep work out of your bedroom; finish up any computer work, Web browsing, or games you play on your device in another room.

BRAIN HEALTH ACTION PLAN

- ☐ Commit to not checking email or social media for a half hour after you awaken.
- ☐ The following week, increase to waiting an hour to check email or social media.

Try nighttime relaxation techniques

- ☐ Try box breathing or 4-7-8 relaxation breathing. Start with 10 rounds and work up to 10 minutes as you feel more comfortable with the practice.
- ☐ Add meditation or prayer.

Foster a healthy circadian rhythm in the daytime

- ☐ Get exposure to bright outside light for 15 minutes within the first 3 hours of the day.
- ☐ If your environment is not conducive to this, consider purchasing a 10,000 lux light box.

Reassess your sleep

- ☐ Use technology to track your sleep to be sure you are getting enough total sleep as well as adequate REM and deep sleep.
- ☐ If you still have room for improvement after optimizing sleep hygiene, ask your doctor if a sleep supplement is appropriate for you.
- ☐ If you take an OTC or prescription medication for sleep, make an appointment with your doctor to discuss the effects and determine if it's still the most appropriate choice for you at your age.

Notes

[1] Lulu Xie, Hongyi Kang, Qiwu Xu, et al., "Sleep drives metabolite clearance from the adult brain," Science 342, no. 6156 (October 2013):373–7, https://doi.org/10.1126%2Fscience.1241224.

[2] Ian M. Colrain, Christian L. Nicholas, Fiona C. Baker, "Alcohol and the sleeping brain," Handb Clin Neurol 125 (2014):415–31, https://doi.org/10.1016%2FB978-0-444-62619-6.00024-0.

[3] Daniel P. Cardinali, "Melatonin: Clinical Perspectives in Neurodegeneration," Front Endocrinol (Lausanne) 10 (July 2019):480, https://doi.org/10.3389/fendo.2019.00480.

[4] Arman Arab, Nahid Rafie, Reza Amani, and Fatemeh Shirani, "The Role of Magnesium in Sleep Health: a Systematic Review of Available Literature," Biol Trace Elem Res 201, no. 1 (January 2023):121–128, https://doi.org/10.1007/s12011-022-03162-1.

[5] Khashayar Farzam, Sarah Sabir, and Maria C. O'Rourke, Antihistamines (Treasure Island, FL: StatPearls Publishing, 2024).

[6] Yo-El S. Ju, Margaret A. Zangrilli, Mary Beth Finn, Anne M. Fagan, and David M. Holtzman, "Obstructive sleep apnea treatment, slow wave activity, and amyloid-β," Ann Neurol. 85, no. 2 (February 2019):291–295, https://doi.org/10.1002/ana.25408.

[7] Mariana Fernandes, Fabio Placidi, Nicola Biagio Mercuri, and Claudio Liguori, "The Importance of Diagnosing and the Clinical Potential of Treating Obstructive Sleep Apnea to Delay Mild Cognitive Impairment and Alzheimer's Disease: A Special Focus on Cognitive Performance," J Alzheimers Dis Rep. 5, no. 1 (June 2021):515–533, https://doi.org/10.3233/ADR-210004.

CHAPTER 12

Get Moving

Physical inactivity is consistently cited as one of the most important modifiable risk factors for the development of Alzheimer's disease. Being sedentary increases inflammation, impairs sugar processing, and increases risk of dementia by 30%.[1] Two-thirds of middle-aged folks are living a sedentary lifestyle. Unfortunately, activity continues to decline with age. In the US, people over eighty are sedentary for an average of nine hours per day![2]

The antidote for inactivity is movement. Studies that examine the link between physical exercise and brain health affirm its benefits. In most studies, this positive effect of exercise on brain health was stronger than with any other intervention. As a result, exercise is the World Health Organization's number-one recommendation for reducing the risk of cognitive decline and dementia.

> *"Physical activity should be recommended to adults with normal cognition to reduce the risk of cognitive decline."*
> —The World Health Organization

The brain thrives with a combination of both **aerobic** (cardio) and **anaerobic** (resistance or strength training) exercise. Both types are consistently linked to enhanced cognitive function and reduced risk of Alzheimer's disease. They exert their beneficial effects through different mechanisms.

Aerobic activities—like running, cycling, or swimming—boost heart rate and blood circulation. Enhanced blood flow increases delivery of oxygen and nutrients that benefit the brain and also helps clear toxins from it.

Anaerobic activities—like weightlifting, strength training, and calisthenics (think jumping jacks, lunges, squats, and push-ups)—target building and maintaining muscle mass. Adequate muscle mass decreases inflammation and helps maintain insulin sensitivity,[3] both of which promote brain health.

Aerobic and anaerobic exercise also provides meaningful brain benefits by triggering the release of myokines.

Myokines are signaling molecules that your muscles make and release into your bloodstream when you exercise. They travel in your bloodstream and play a role in communication between your muscles and other organ systems. Myokines influence metabolism, immune function, inflammation, and even brain health.[4]

Brain-derived neurotrophic factor (BDNF) is a myokine that deserves special attention because it is a key factor in preserving brain health and function. BDNF supports the growth of new neurons in the hippocampus, helps protect your existing neurons from damage, strengthens synaptic connections between neurons, and is directly involved in learning, forming memories, and problem-solving.[5] It's also involved in mood regulation and mental health, which we'll cover in Chapter 15.

Brain Improvement You Can Measure

Strength training affects the brain in positive and measurable ways. We know that Alzheimer's disease shrinks the brain's short-term memory structures called the hippocampi. The left hippocampus usually shrinks more than the right. Amazingly, a 2020 study showed that doing resistance training exercise for ninety minutes two to three times per week for six months protected the left hippocampus from shrinkage.[6]

No doubt about it: physical inactivity is the most important modifiable risk factor to tackle if you're interested in staving off dementia. If you're not already exercising, figuring out how to incorporate movement in your lifestyle-based dementia risk-reduction plan can be daunting. Where to start? How much exercise do you need? What type of exercise? And what if you hate it?

Read on.

Which Exercise Is Best?

Most research on exercise's impact on brain health focuses on walking because it's easy to standardize, easy to measure, and widely available. But the abundance of research that illustrates how walking helps keep your brain healthy should not be misinterpreted as saying it's the best or only exercise for accomplishing that goal. Walking, running, swimming, dancing, and cycling are all good options for heart-rate-boosting aerobic activity, while resistance training, weightlifting, and calisthenics offer the benefits of anaerobic exercises.

There isn't an exercise regimen that's best for everyone. The best type of exercise for you is the type you can do and will do. As you search for movement that meets those two criteria, try to incorporate a combination of both aerobic and anaerobic exercises so you can harness each of their brain-boosting benefits.

Tale of a Hypocritical Neurologist

In 2015, I preached the benefits of exercise to my patients every day. I encouraged them to start or increase their exercise and helped them track their progress.

Meanwhile, I wasn't exercising.

Like so many people, I just didn't enjoy it. I also didn't think I had time to exercise. A seemingly little thing finally pierced the veil of my hypocrisy: one day, I struggled to pick up a box that shouldn't have been a challenge for me. I was shocked to realize that I was losing strength. Of all people, I knew the terrible effects that loss of muscle mass and lack of exercise could have on my brain, and I knew I had to change.

I started by joining my husband on his daily dog walks around our neighborhood. I felt great after walking. After several months of walking daily, I actually *wanted* to exercise more, so I started taking exercise classes. Everyone in my family participates in CrossFit, and my husband is even a CrossFit instructor. So, naturally, I started with that. But it wasn't a good fit for me. Even though my family members are in wonderful shape and I knew it would be great for my brain and body, I couldn't force myself to do exercise I disliked. I tried all kinds of classes offered at the Y, through my city, and at a local gym. I finally discovered Pilates, and I love it!

Here's the moral of the story: If I can adopt a new exercise habit, I bet you can too! Start small, and keep trying new exercises until you find one you enjoy.

How Much Exercise?

The ultimate goal for reducing the risk of Alzheimer's disease is doing a combination of aerobic and anaerobic exercise **twenty to forty-five minutes per day, at least five days a week.**

To the readers who are thinking, *There is no way! There is absolutely no way I'm going to find the time, energy, or desire to accomplish that much exercise*, please don't put down this book. We're going to incorporate mini habits so you can start exercising with minimal time and energy. You're going to start with the most miniature habit you can think of. Can you set a goal to do one squat every day? Or walk for one minute? It may sound ridiculous, but that accomplishment builds momentum and helps reestablish a healthy relationship with exercise. You can choose any kind of movement you enjoy. You should feel good after you exercise; you don't have to hurt or sweat to reap its brain health benefits. If you think of exercise as punishment, it's time to reframe exercise as movement and understand that it is a generous form of self-care. **Exercise is the most effective way to keep your brain healthy**, and there simply isn't another way to harness its benefits.

For readers who already exercise but aren't quite at the goal level mentioned, your path will look a bit different. When you get to this chapter's goals and mini habits, find the level of exercise that meets you where you are. Use mini goals to tweak your regimen to optimize the duration of your exercise, and be sure it includes both aerobic and anaerobic exercise.

Last, for **folks who love to exercise** and are already meeting or exceeding the recommendation above, congratulations! Your work here is done. Skip to the next chapter.

Starting from Scratch? Build Your Exercise Habit Gradually.

If you're starting from scratch and don't already have an exercise in mind, think of a time when you did exercise. Did you enjoy it? If you did, could you start again?

If nothing comes to mind or you can't restart an exercise you once enjoyed, start with the first step in the list of mini habits at the end of the chapter. That's a one-minute daily walk or one calisthenic, like a squat, lunge, jumping jack, or modified push-up. Each week, slightly increase the duration of your walk or add to the number of calisthenics you do. Once you have built a good exercise baseline of walking and calisthenics, consider branching out and exploring other types of exercise, like taking group classes or working with a trainer to see if you can find anything else you enjoy.

As you build your exercise habit, be sure to include both aerobic and anaerobic activities. Brisk walking, running, bicycling, and swimming count as aerobic activity, which increases heart rate and healthy blood flow to the brain. Lifting weights, using resistance bands, and doing calisthenics are examples of anaerobic exercise that will build muscle and supercharge your myokine release. If balance is an issue, do lunges and squats holding onto a chair or counter for support; modify push-ups by doing them more vertically by pushing up against a table or counter rather than horizontally on the floor.

Leveling up your exercise will mean different things to different people based on ability. For example, if you're walking forty-five minutes several times a week and want to continue to push yourself, you could walk longer or spend part of that time running instead of walking. However, devoting more time to exercise may not be realistic. Similarly, running may not be realistic for many folks. Instead, you might consider wearing wrist or ankle weights while you walk or converting your walk into a "ruck" by wearing a weight vest. Rucking adds resistance exercise to your walk and can help you maintain posture, build muscle mass, and improve bone density. Consult your medical provider to determine if adding weight to your walk is appropriate for you.

> **Does Walking Your Dog Count as Exercise?**
>
> It depends on how vigorous the walk is. If your dog visits every tree, you're probably not achieving a pace of walking that gives your body and brain the exercise benefit you deserve. If your dog is keeping pace with you and does not stop often, you may be getting adequate exercise.
>
> The American Heart Association can also help you answer this question. Head to the AHA website, www.heart.org, and search "Target Heart Rates Chart." You can measure your heart rate at the end of your walk and see if you are reaching the target rate zone for exercise for your age group.
>
> If you aren't getting your heart rate to the target zone with your dog walk, it still presents an excellent opportunity to build your exercise habit. Take a walk with the dog, then drop Fido off at home, and go for a brief, vigorous walk alone. Since you are already in walking shoes and comfortable clothes and you're not likely to let your furry friend down by ignoring their need for a walk, this can be a great way to stack habits.

Take Action: Tasks, Goals, and Mini Habits

Assess your readiness

- ☐ If you're feeling intimidated by starting to exercise, spend a few minutes thinking about the benefits of keeping your brain healthy.

- [ ] If you're going to need to build a lot of new mini habits, consider rereading Chapter 4 to review how to set effective goals.

- [ ] Put pen to paper. Brainstorm exercises that you enjoy and new exercises you might consider. What have you tried in the past? Why did you discontinue?

- [ ] If you are noticing some resistance to starting exercise, skip to a chapter where you can get some easy wins in developing new habits and ride that wave of success back to this chapter with fresh eyes.

Gradually build an exercise habit that supports optimal brain health

Your exercise tasks and habits are likely to require a lot of customization since we are all starting at a different baseline and have different preferences and abilities. Find the level below that fits you, check off all the previous levels, and go from there. Each task should be a 1-to-2-week streak.

- [ ] Walk daily for 1 minute.
- [ ] Walk daily for 1 minute, followed by one calisthenic (a squat, lunge, jumping jack, modified push-up, etc.).
- [ ] Walk daily for 5 minutes, followed by 5 calisthenics.
- [ ] Walk daily for 10 minutes, followed by 5 calisthenics.

BRAIN HEALTH ACTION PLAN

☐ Walk daily for 15 minutes, followed by 5 calisthenics.

☐ Walk daily for 20 minutes, followed by 10 calisthenics (consider incorporating a couple of different types of calisthenics to move different parts of your body).

☐ Walk daily for 25 minutes, followed by 10 calisthenics.

☐ Walk daily for 30 minutes, followed by 10 calisthenics.

☐ Walk daily for 30 minutes, and add mid-walk calisthenics, like 5 squats or lunges at every corner (if your balance allows you to do so safely), followed by 10 more calisthenics when you return home.

☐ Walk daily for 35 minutes, doing 5 mid-walk calisthenics and 10 post-walk calisthenics.

☐ Walk daily for 40 minutes, doing 5 mid-walk calisthenics and 10 post-walk calisthenics.

☐ Walk daily for 40 minutes, doing 5 mid-walk calisthenics and 15 post-walk calisthenics.

☐ Walk daily for 45 minutes, doing 10 mid-walk calisthenics and 15 post-walk calisthenics.

☐ Identify another time when you can add 5 more calisthenics to your day. Habit stack these to another activity. For example, prior to showering, every time you get up from the computer, etc.

Branch out and level up

- ☐ Check your local parks and recreation department or local gyms and exercise businesses for exercise class schedules.
- ☐ Consider using an app like ClassPass (www.classpass.com) to find local exercise classes. It's a great way to experiment!
- ☐ Level up your walk by adding weight—either limb weights or a weight vest to make it a "ruck." Consult your physician to determine the appropriate weight for your body and health situation.

Personalize your exercise regimen

- ☐ If the above lists don't align with exercises you like and can do, write down your current exercise or an exercise you can do, and plan to start with that. Each week, when you set your next exercise mini goal, increase one variable: distance, speed, duration, repetitions, weight, sessions, etc.

Notes

[1] Shihiao Yan, Wenning Fu, Chao Wang, et al., "Association between sedentary behavior and the risk of dementia: a systematic review and meta-analysis," Transl Psych 10 (2020):110, https://doi.org/10.1 038%2Fs41398-020-0799-5.

[2] Shoshanna Vaynman and Fernando Gomez-Pinilla, "Revenge of the 'sit': how lifestyle impacts neuronal and cognitive health through molecular systems that interface energy metabolism with neuronal plasticity," J Neurosci Res 84, no. 4 (September 2006):699–715, https://doi.org/10.1002/jnr.20979.

[3] Samad Esmaeilzadeh, Susanne Kumpulainen, Arto J. Pesola, "Strength-Cognitive Training: A Systemic Review in Adults and Older Adults, and Guidelines to Promote 'Strength Exergaming' Innovations," Front Psychol 13 (May 2022):855703, https://doi.org/10.3389/fpsyg.2022.855703.

[4] Alessandra Pratesi, Francesca Tarantini, and Mauro Di Bari, "Skeletal muscle: an endocrine organ," Clin Cases Miner Bone Metab 10, no. 1 (January 2013):11–4, https://doi.org/10.11138/ccmbm/2013.10.1.011.

[5] Sujin Kim, Ji-Young Choi, Sohee Moon, Dong-Ho Park, Hyo-Bum Kwak, and Ju-Hee Kang, "Roles of myokines in exercise-induced improvement of neuropsychiatric function," Pflugers Arch 471, no. 3 (March 2019):491–505, https://doi.org/10.1007/s00424-019-02253-8.

[6] Kathryn M. Broadhouse, Maria Fiatarone Singh, et al., "Hippocampal plasticity underpins long-term cognitive gains from resistance exercise in MCI," Neuroimage Clin 25 (2020):102182, https://doi.org/10.1016/j.nicl.2020.102182.

CHAPTER 13

Education and Exercising Your Brain

Your Brain throughout Your Life Cycle

When you were born, your brain had about 100 billion neurons! That was just about all the neurons you would ever have. Throughout childhood, your brain matured and created new connections until it reached its maximum size in early adulthood. From that point on, you've been gradually losing brain cells. In fact, between the ages of thirty and seventy, you will lose 10% of your brain.

Scientists once thought the adult human brain couldn't grow new neurons. But in 1998, Swedish researchers surprised the world with their discovery that the brain does make new cells in a process called neurogenesis.[1] They were able to identify new, young cells in the hippocampus on autopsy of individuals up to age seventy-five. This was great news for people who were trying to increase cognitive reserve and stave off Alzheimer's disease.

Understanding how new neurons grow and connect can help us develop lifestyle habits that nurture their survival. When a new neuron develops, it is like a shrub with branches reaching out in many directions, trying to form connections—synapses—with other neurons. When you engage in learning and other brain-stimulating exercises, the new neuron's branches start communicating with other neurons. Eventually, they form a durable synaptic connection with other neurons and join the vast communication networks in your brain.

If your brain grows a new memory neuron in the hippocampus but you aren't challenging your brain with complex thoughts and new learning, that neuron's branches won't form durable synapses with other neurons. The unconnected branches serve no purpose and will activate a process called synaptic pruning. This brain maintenance process comes through and chops off the neuronal branches that failed to make a connection, much like you might prune leafless branches from a shrub. If the neuron made no connections, it will be pruned to nothingness.

Education and Lifelong Learning

Low education is high on the list of modifiable risk factors for Alzheimer's disease.

> "I didn't finish high school. Is it too late? Do I have to go back to school?"

The good news is no; you don't have to go back to school. Education is not limited to formal schooling. If a person who didn't finish high school embraces lifelong learning, they have the same chance of great brain health as someone who has a graduate degree. No matter how far you went in school, brain exercise can improve this risk factor.

When you challenge your brain with complex tasks, you increase blood flow to it. This delivers healthy nutrients and washes away toxins. Spending years in school isn't the only way to do that. Complex work stimulates the same healthy blood flow. So does creativity. There are so many ways to harness the advantage of learning that is often oversimplified with the word *education*. It's not the years you spent in formal education that keep your brain healthy. It's the amount of time you spend thinking hard and solving problems that accomplishes this goal.

"I have two graduate degrees, so this risk factor doesn't apply to me."

I don't recommend resting on the laurels of higher education. Advances in the understanding of neurogenesis demonstrate how important it is to continue learning throughout our lifetime. Keep challenging your brain with new information so that you head into your senior years with as much cognitive reserve as possible.

> *"An uneducated but mentally active individual has the same opportunity of lessening the risk of Alzheimer's as an Oxford don."*
> —Jack C. de la Torre, Alzheimer's Turning Point, *2016*

Cognitive Reserve

Cognitive reserve is like a backup reservoir of neurons that you can access in case of emergency. High cognitive reserve means having plentiful brain tissue and extensive connections within it. Having more brain cells with more connections means that if you have damage in one brain pathway, you can compensate by using another brain pathway.

The ninety-plus study[2] conducted in Laguna Woods, California, confirmed the significance of cognitive reserve. Scientists looked at the brains of previously healthy nonagenarians (people in their nineties) and were surprised to find some of their brains contained extensive signs of Alzheimer's disease. How could these folks accumulate so much brain disease without experiencing cognitive decline or dementia? The answer is that they had built high cognitive reserve through education, complex work, and leisure activities. Their cognitive reserve allowed them to continue to live a full and independent lifestyle using alternative brain pathways to get around diseased areas.

Cognitive Exercise

It is a fact that those people who demand more of their brains during their lifetime are able to maintain a higher volume of cells in their hippocampal memory centers. Work is generally a cognitively complex activity, and that is probably why people who delay retirement have better cognitive function later in life than those who voluntarily retire early. If you are working, your endeavors are cognitive exercise, so you may not have to devote as much time to after-work cognitive exercise for cognitive exercise's sake.

If you are no longer working in a formal capacity, it's a good idea to set up a brain exercise regimen, just like you would set goals for physical exercise. Games are a great place to start. People tend to play mental games that draw on their cognitive talents while avoiding games that rely on mental skills that aren't as well-developed. People who love crossword puzzles can easily build a brain-healthy habit of doing them daily. The same can be said for people who love reading, sudoku, or Wordle. They're all cognitively stimulating, but each one exercises only a couple of specific areas of the brain. Your goal is to exercise your whole brain. You have many different cognitive functions and structures, so any you neglect to exercise are at risk of becoming weak. It's a lot like your body and physical exercise. Let's imagine you went to the gym every day and focused only on biceps curls. The upshot, of course, is you would have rocking biceps! Unfortunately, though, that would leave the rest of your body weak. Just as you must exercise all parts of your body to keep it strong, so must you exercise all parts of your brain.

If you have a brain game you enjoy, that's fantastic! Keep playing it daily and build a regimen to exercise the other parts of your brain too. Designing such a regimen on your own can be intimidating and time-consuming, and you might not know what activities to add to exercise all parts of your brain. Thankfully, cognitive training programs have addressed this challenge.

Boot Camp for Your Brain

BrainHQ and Lumosity are two examples of brain exercise programs that you can use on your computer or smartphone. These programs run you through a bunch of different brain games that stimulate different brain regions in a short period of time. They also track your progress. Brain training ideally should be done daily. Some even have a built-in streak tracker that shows how many days in a row you have done your daily cognitive exercise.

If you prefer pen-and-paper tasks, there are workbooks that exercise your brain in many areas. These take a bit more time, and it's not as easy to track your progress as it is with online versions.

Games

Playing games with an opponent is another way to exercise your brain. The more cognitively demanding the game, the better. Bridge and chess, for example, simultaneously exercise multiple parts of your brain that are involved in logic, problem-solving, pattern recognition, memory, and spatial reasoning.

New, Fun, and Effective: Neurobics

Neurobics are mental gymnastics that help maintain mental flexibility, processing speed, and memory. These brain-stretching exercises use one of your brain processes—language, movement, hearing, vision, taste, or smell—in an atypical way or combine two different processes in an unusual way. You can challenge your brain by doing familiar tasks in an unfamiliar way. For example, you might brush your teeth or write with your nondominant hand, or take a new route home. Try wearing your watch upside down so your brain must work harder to tell the time. To experiment with neurobics that combine two brain processes, try walking upstairs while counting down from a hundred by fives, or gather several different spices, close your eyes, and try to identify each by smell. Then, keeping your eyes closed, spell the name of the spice out loud, forward and backward.

Take a Class

Your daily cognitive exercise program—online, app based, or a workbook—is a great baseline brain health habit, but don't stop there. Take a class to stimulate new learning. Indulge your creativity and curiosity, and find something that interests you. It could be learning a new language, picking up an instrument you used to play, taking an art class or history class, or finally signing up to learn how to do something you've been interested in. The course can be online or in person. You can even decide to learn a new skill by watching lessons on YouTube.

Take Action: Tasks, Goals, and Mini Habits

Do daily cognitive exercise and seek opportunities for new learning

- ☐ Write down all the things you do on a daily basis that give your brain a workout.

- ☐ Brainstorm games and cognitive activities you enjoy and could do more of. Some examples are reading, crossword puzzles, sudoku, bridge, cards, backgammon, chess, and classes.

- ☐ Sign up for an online daily cognitive exercise program app like BrainHQ or Lumosity, or purchase a cognitive exercise workbook.

- ☐ Add a cognitive exercise you already like from your brainstorm list. If, for example, you like sudoku, order a workbook or download an app so you can do sudoku puzzles daily after your brain is warmed up with your online cognitive exercise program or cognitive exercise workbook.

- ☐ Check out the class schedules for your city's parks and recreation department, local centers, or local community college for interesting classes you can take.

- ☐ Play a game at least once per week. If finding a partner is difficult, consider playing chess, backgammon, or bridge online.

- ☐ Download a list of neurobics and choose a different one to do each day.

Notes

[1] Eriksson PS, Perfilieva E, Björk-Eriksson T, Alborn AM, Nordborg C, Peterson DA, Gage FH, "Neurogenesis in the adult human hippocampus," Nat Med. 4, no. 11 (November 1998):1313–7, https://doi.org/10.1038/3305.

[2] Claudia H. Kawas, Ronald C. Kim, Joshua A. Sonnen, Szofia S. Bullain, Thomas Trieu, and María M. Corrada, "Multiple pathologies are common and related to dementia in the oldest-old: The 90+ Study," Neurology 85, no. 6 (August 2015):535–42, https://doi.org/10.1212/WNL.0000000000001831.

CHAPTER 14

How General Health Affects Brain Health

Every organ system has an important role to play in your overall health, and the health of each organ is tied to brain health. In fact, sometimes the brain acts as the canary in the coal mine, signaling the presence of an undiagnosed general medical problem. That's because the brain requires a near-perfect environment to function well.

So far, we have focused on maintaining a healthy lifestyle to lessen the risk of Alzheimer's disease. This chapter will focus on the importance of working with your health care provider to identify underlying conditions or effectively treat chronic diseases that can cause brain dysfunction.

Because the brain is such a sensitive organ, changes in blood nutrients, toxins, hormones, and oxygen levels can impair brain function. **Encephalopathy** is the medical term for brain dysfunction and encompasses a wide variety of symptoms from confusion and memory loss to coma.

There are many different causes of encephalopathy, so it makes sense to break them down into categories.

Degenerative encephalopathies are brain diseases that cause neuron degeneration and death, like Alzheimer's disease.

Metabolic encephalopathies arise from metabolic imbalances in the body. For example, when the liver or kidneys aren't working well, toxins build up in the blood that can impair normal brain function. Electrolyte imbalance, vitamin deficiencies, thyroid problems, and high or low sugar levels are all metabolic causes of encephalopathy.

Exposing the brain to medications, drugs, alcohol, and other substances that directly affect brain function can cause **toxic encephalopathy**. Medications that can cause encephalopathy are discussed in this chapter, and other toxins are discussed in Chapter 16.

When viruses, bacteria, or fungi directly infect the brain, those are called **infectious encephalopathies**. Some examples include Herpes encephalitis, West Nile encephalitis, and neurologic Lyme disease.

When the cardiovascular system isn't delivering adequate blood and oxygen to the brain, that's called **hypoxic-ischemic encephalopathy**. That might occur as a result of a stroke or heart attack. Another example of brain dysfunction due to problems in the cardiovascular system is when severe hypertension (high blood pressure) goes unchecked. Severe hypertension can cause brain swelling and lead to confusion and even coma. It is called **hypertensive encephalopathy**.

Last, physical trauma to the brain can cause **traumatic encephalopathy**.

Staying current on annual visits to your physician for health screening and lab work is an effective way to identify medical problems before they cause brain symptoms. Let's discuss the areas that you and your provider can address to avoid encephalopathy.

Hydration

Dehydration and overhydration can both lead to brain dysfunction. Dehydration becomes more prevalent as we age and is a common cause of confusion in seniors. However, even with something as important as water, you can have too much of a good thing. Massive water intake leads to overhydration or "water intoxication." Water intoxication dilutes salt and other electrolytes in your blood, which can lead to brain swelling and even death. Although dehydration is a more common problem than water intoxication, it's a good reminder that moderation is usually the right approach for health resolutions. If you've strayed away from your healthy hydration habit, consider revisiting Chapter 6.

Electrolyte Abnormalities

Electrolytes are ions and electrically charged minerals that play a crucial role in functions throughout the brain and body. Common electrolytes include sodium, calcium, potassium, and magnesium.

Electrolytes are essential for maintaining proper fluid balance, conducting electrical impulses, and supporting cell and organ function. They are particularly important for brain function due to their involvement in nerve transmission and communication between neurons. Small shifts in electrolytes can cause big changes in brain function.

Brain cells rely on the difference between electrolyte concentrations outside and inside cells to generate electricity, and that electricity is how the nervous system communicates and transmits signals. Normal thinking, focus, and memory rely on proper brain electrolyte balance.

Improper intake of water or electrolytes can disrupt the delicate balance of electrolytes in the brain. In rare cases, electrolyte imbalance becomes severe, leading to confusion, memory loss, and other neurological problems, like seizures. The following table lists some of the symptoms that people can experience with severe shifts in sodium, calcium, potassium, and magnesium:

Electrolyte Abnormality	Neurologic Symptoms
Low sodium	Headache, lethargy, seizures
High sodium	Weakness, tremor, encephalopathy
Low calcium	Numbness, tingling, confusion, psychosis
High calcium	Weakness, depression, dementia, anxiety
Low potassium	Weakness, leg cramps, muscle breakdown
Low magnesium	Tremor, headache, confusion
High magnesium	Weakness

Vascular Conditions

The term *vascular* refers to your arteries and veins—the vital structures that carry blood throughout the body. Hypertension, high cholesterol, diabetes, and smoking can damage the arteries that supply blood to your organs. When that process affects the arteries that deliver blood to the brain, it's called cerebrovascular disease (*cerebro* = brain; *vascular* = blood vessels). Cerebrovascular disease increases the risk of stroke and dementia. Managing these risk factors is a cornerstone of protecting brain health.

Atherosclerosis

What do your arteries and the slimy outer layer of fish have in common? Both have a protective layer called glycocalyx.

The glycocalyx is slippery. In fish, it provides a protective barrier against infections and reduces friction as fish swim through the water. Glycocalyx functions similarly in your arteries. It provides a protective barrier against toxins and infections and reduces friction as the blood cells travel through blood vessels. This slippery layer acts like a Teflon coating that prevents blood and its contents from sticking to the sides of the artery walls.

Several factors can damage the delicate glycocalyx—our familiar foes, hypertension, high blood sugar, smoking, and chronic inflammation.[1] When the glycocalyx is damaged or inflamed, white blood cells, red blood cells, and cholesterol stick to that area. From there, they migrate into the artery wall and form a plaque. This results in narrowing and hardening of the arteries, called **atherosclerosis**. Atherosclerosis in the cerebral arteries results in decreased blood flow to the brain. When this process blocks an artery in the brain, it can cause a transient ischemic attack (TIA) or stroke. When atherosclerosis lessens flow to tiny capillary blood vessels in the brain, there might not be an immediate symptom that indicates that a tiny part of the brain is starved for blood. However, over time, the cumulative effect of inadequate blood flow to the capillaries becomes apparent, resulting in slow movement, slow thinking, and eventually dementia.

Exercising and eating an antioxidant-rich, low-sugar diet are lifestyle choices that lessen inflammation to keep your glycocalyx healthy. Scientists have discovered seaweed's potential ability to protect the glycocalyx. In animal studies, a seaweed-derived compound called rhamnan sulfate improves glycocalyx health and reduces atherosclerosis.[2] Not only does rhamnan sulfate have anti-inflammatory and antioxidant properties, it also may reduce "bad" LDL cholesterol.[3]

Hypertension

Hypertension is the medical term for high blood pressure. It means that the blood pressure in the arteries is high, which damages them and the protective blood-brain barrier (BBB). When the BBB is compromised, toxins can access the brain more easily. Furthermore, uncontrolled hypertension also boosts brain inflammation and beta-amyloid deposition—known to be a basic pathway to Alzheimer's disease.[4]

How important is treating hypertension? The Lancet Commission on Dementia Prevention declared that medications used to treat hypertension are "the only known effective prevention medication for dementia."[5]

In addition to taking medications that alleviate high blood pressure, eating well, sleeping well, exercising, and meditating are lifestyle habits that can also help reduce hypertension. Drinking alcohol can also affect blood pressure. A 2017 study[6] published in *The Lancet* found that lowering alcohol intake often lessens hypertension. Interestingly, this pattern was seen only in hypertensive people who usually drank more than two alcoholic beverages daily. People with hypertension who consumed one to two alcoholic beverages daily did not see an improvement in blood pressure when they lowered their alcohol intake.

Diabetes

People with diabetes have high levels of sugar in the blood. As excess sugar travels in the bloodstream, it attaches to glycocalyx and to the structural proteins in the artery walls. Sugar-laden glycocalyx loses its ability to protect artery walls from toxins and infections, triggers inflammation, and becomes sticky. Structural proteins covered with sugar molecules aren't able to perform their job of adjusting blood flow according to the body's needs, making the system less responsive. Together, these processes impair proper blood flow and contribute to the development of atherosclerosis.

High Cholesterol

Cholesterol is a fatty substance that is essential for cell structure and hormone production. The brain contains a significant amount of cholesterol, and brain cells couldn't function without it. However, having high levels of cholesterol in the blood, particularly low-density lipoprotein (LDL) cholesterol, is a risk factor for cerebrovascular disease.

Cholesterol is a key player in the formation of atherosclerotic plaques that contribute to brain disease and cognitive impairment. The American Heart Association (AHA) recommends cholesterol screening as part of routine health assessments starting at age twenty. When high cholesterol is identified, providers often recommend lifestyle-centered approaches, such as following the Mediterranean diet and increasing exercise, as the first step in trying to reduce it. Medications or supplements may be necessary if lifestyle adjustments don't yield the desired improvement.

Smoking

Smoking aggressively damages cerebral arteries and accelerates atherosclerosis through multiple mechanisms, including inflammation of the glycocalyx. Although smoking cessation is beyond the scope of this book, you can read more about its brain health consequences in Chapter 16 and consult your physician for advice when you decide to quit.

Thyroid Dysfunction

The thyroid gland is a small butterfly-shaped organ located at the base of the neck, below the Adam's apple. It produces hormones that regulate metabolism throughout the body, including metabolism and energy production in the brain. Thyroid hormones also modulate the production and activity of neurotransmitters, such as serotonin, dopamine, GABA, and norepinephrine. According to the American Thyroid Association, about twenty million Americans suffer from thyroid disease, and about half of them are unaware of their condition.

Underactive Thyroid

Hypothyroidism is an underactive thyroid gland that doesn't produce enough thyroid hormones. If your thyroid isn't working well, your metabolism will be slow and you'll feel tired. Low thyroid also suppresses brain metabolism and creates neurotransmitter imbalance, which can lead to slow thinking, confusion, poor memory, and depression.

The symptoms of hypothyroidism can be subtle and non-specific, so it often goes undiagnosed until screening labs are done. When underactive thyroid is treated early, the brain goes back to normal. If diagnosis and treatment of underactive thyroid is severely delayed, it can lead to permanent changes in brain function. It's important to follow your doctor's recommendation for routine thyroid lab screening.

Overactive Thyroid

An overactive thyroid, called hyperthyroidism, can also cause neurological symptoms. Overproduction of thyroid hormones sends metabolism into overdrive, causing rapid heartbeat, tremors, weight loss, and heat intolerance. It also overstimulates the nervous system, leading to anxiety, irritability, and confusion. These symptoms are much more noticeable than those of hypothyroidism, often leading to earlier diagnosis. The neurological symptoms related to overactive thyroid usually resolve completely with medical treatment.

Liver and Kidney Disease

The liver and kidneys are both involved in detoxifying the blood. If they aren't working well, toxins accumulate in the blood. Subsequently, the bloodstream transports these toxins to the brain, resulting in confusion. Severe dysfunction of the liver or kidneys can lead to toxin-induced hallucinations or coma. Regular monitoring of liver and kidney function through routine labs is often part of annual checkups. This helps identify any early changes in function, allowing for timely intervention and prevention of serious complications.

Hearing Loss

Studies show that hearing loss doubles dementia risk.[7] Although we don't know the exact mechanism, scientists have several theories about how hearing loss might contribute to the development of Alzheimer's disease. First, hearing loss can lead to social isolation and difficulty engaging in conversations. Social isolation and loneliness are known risk factors for cognitive impairment. In addition, people with hearing loss may be more prone to depression, which is itself a known risk factor for dementia. Hearing loss may also lead to reduced cognitive reserve, making individuals more vulnerable to the effects of brain aging, as discussed in Chapter 13. Finally, the most common type of hearing loss in aging, which starts in the inner ear, is associated with accelerated shrinkage of the brain. More recently, researchers have answered the obvious next question: does correcting hearing loss reduce that risk? Indeed, it does! A 2022 study revealed that correcting hearing loss with hearing aids or cochlear implants reduced dementia risk by 19% and improved cognitive test scores by 3%.[8]

The average adult with hearing loss waits about nine years to seek treatment. If you or a loved one has noticed that you aren't hearing well, get your hearing tested. This is an important treatable risk factor for dementia. Even if you don't think you have hearing loss, consider a hearing test to establish your baseline, then follow your audiologist's recommendations for repeat screening.

Dental Hygiene

By now, I'm sure you are convinced that what you put in your mouth has important implications for your brain health. But what about how you take care of your mouth?

Researchers studied the brains of people who died from Alzheimer's disease and found bacteria associated with gingivitis (gum inflammation) in almost all of them. These particular bacteria, called *Porphyromonas gingivalis*, can move from the mouth to the brain and are known to release an enzyme that kills nerve cells.

Dental health is important. Brushing, flossing, and keeping up to date with dental visits can help you maintain brain health.

Vitamin Deficiencies

Vitamin B12

Vitamin B12 plays a key role in getting energy from fat, making blood cells, forming DNA, and maintaining the nervous system. Although vitamin B12 deficiency can cause a wide range of symptoms throughout the nervous system, here we'll focus primarily on its cognitive symptoms: memory loss and confusion.

The American diet generally contains adequate vitamin B12, which is found naturally in meat and dairy products. Vitamin B12 deficiency is rarely due to a lack of vitamin B12 in our diet. Rather, deficiency usually arises from the body's inability to process or absorb it from food. Vitamin B12 is processed in the stomach and then absorbed in the small intestine. It's helpful to understand how the body processes and absorbs vitamin B12 so you can see how medications and changes in your gut could lead to deficiency.

> *Strict vegetarians and vegans are at risk of inadequate vitamin B12 intake. If you fit into either group, pay special attention to include nonanimal foods fortified with vitamin B12, and ask your nutritionist or doctor if you should take a vitamin B12 supplement.*

Vitamin B12 is processed in the stomach. Stomach acid releases vitamin B12 from food. Next, a compound called gastric intrinsic factor (IF) binds to the free-floating vitamin B12 and accompanies it on its journey to the small intestine, where it is absorbed. Vitamin B12 must be bound to IF in order for the small intestine to absorb it.

In the stomach, there are several medications that can impede vitamin B12 processing. Medications like omeprazole (Prilosec) and lansoprazole (Prevacid) lessen heartburn from gastroesophageal reflux disease (GERD) by reducing stomach acid. Without enough stomach acid, B12 won't be released from food and cannot undergo any further processing or absorption. Cholestyramine is a medication that lowers cholesterol by binding to it, but cholestyramine can also bind to IF. Last, vitamin C can break down vitamin B12 in the gut before it has a chance to get absorbed. For this reason, it is frequently recommended that vitamin C be taken at least two hours after vitamin B12.

Weight loss surgery, peptic ulcer disease, and inflammation of the stomach, called gastritis, can also decrease or prevent proper vitamin B12 processing in the stomach. Up to 30% of older adults suffer from gastritis, which may be one reason vitamin B12 deficiency increases with age.

Vitamin B12 attached to IF is absorbed in a part of the intestine called the ileum. Medications such as colchicine (Colcrys), metformin (Glucophage), and some antibiotics are known to interfere with vitamin B12 absorption. Antibiotics and the anti-inflammatory medication colchicine are usually taken for a short time, so their temporary decrease in vitamin B12 absorption is unlikely to cause vitamin B12 deficiency. Metformin, on the other hand, is used to treat diabetes and may be taken for years. Studies show that the likelihood of developing a vitamin B12 deficiency increases with the duration of metformin use. Millions of people take this medication. Doctors usually monitor vitamin B12 levels once patients have been on it for several years.

Physical changes in the small intestine that can reduce vitamin B12 absorption include celiac disease, Crohn's disease, small intestine bacterial overgrowth (SIBO), small intestine surgery, and infestations. Celiac disease and Crohn's disease are both characterized by inflammation of and damage to the intestinal lining, which knocks out its ability to absorb vitamin B12. SIBO and infestations prevent vitamin B12 absorption in a different way. When the small intestine gets overpopulated with bacteria, these bacteria steal vitamin B12 for their own use before it can be absorbed. Bacteria aren't the only scavengers that divert vitamin B12. Although parasitic infestations are relatively uncommon in the US, tapeworms in the small intestine can siphon off nutrients, including vitamin B12, to use for their own growth.

Speak with your doctor about measuring your vitamin B12 level if you have any of the following risk factors: vegan or strict vegetarian, age >50, history of gut surgery, taking any of the medications listed above, one of the digestive conditions mentioned above, or a first-degree relative with celiac disease.

Vitamin D

Vitamin D is often called the sunshine vitamin because our bodies produce it in our skin in response to sunlight. When your skin thins in midlife, you absorb about half of the vitamin D you did earlier in life. Vitamin D can also be absorbed from food and is found in fish, eggs, and mushrooms. Unfortunately, you'd have to eat a dozen eggs a day to meet your daily vitamin D requirement.

Vitamin D is technically a hormone that has a wide range of effects throughout the body. In addition to its familiar role in bone health, vitamin D is recognized for its neuroprotective properties. It is anti-inflammatory[9] and reduces amyloid and tau in laboratory studies.[10]

Vitamin D deficiency is linked to an increased risk of Alzheimer's disease.[11] Fortunately, studies also show that taking a vitamin D supplement can reduce the risk of Alzheimer's disease.[12] For this reason, maintaining normal vitamin D levels should be part of your brain health action plan. Be sure to discuss vitamin D screening with your medical provider.

Hormones

Whether you are male or female, your brain is covered with receptors for estrogen and testosterone. These hormones have a complex relationship with brain health, and hormone balance is necessary for optimal brain function.

Shifts in hormone levels throughout your lifespan influence cognitive performance as well as risk of neurodegenerative diseases such as Alzheimer's disease.[13]

Estrogen and testosterone have a great deal in common. They are both neuroprotective, meaning they support the growth and survival of neurons. They have antioxidant and anti-inflammatory properties that help derail two of the core processes of Alzheimer's disease. They also increase BDNF—the compound discussed in Chapter 12 that helps nerve cells in your brain grow, adapt, and survive.

These hormones also influence mood, behavior, and memory by regulating three neurotransmitters that brain cells use to communicate with each other: acetylcholine, serotonin, and dopamine.

Menopause

Radical shifts in hormones during menopause commonly lead to brain fog. This phenomenon does not surprise neuroscientists, and now that you understand the influence of hormones on your brain, it probably doesn't surprise you either. Whether or not premenopausal levels of hormones should be restored in postmenopausal women has been and continues to be the subject of much research, debate, and spirited discussion.[14]

Over the past several decades, hormone replacement therapy (HRT) guidelines have evolved significantly. In the 1970s, HRT was hailed for its potential ability to protect against heart disease and was almost universally recommended to postmenopausal women. Then, in the early 2000s, a large study called the Women's Health Initiative[15] raised concerns that HRT might actually *increase* heart disease and other disorders. HRT guidelines changed virtually overnight. Millions of postmenopausal women were taken off HRT, and millions more were not started on HRT in the following twenty years. Subsequent research has helped clarify how factors like age, timing of initiation of HRT, duration of use, and formulation of hormones might influence the risks and benefits.[16] As a result, the guidelines are again shifting—this time from universal discouragement of HRT to an individualized approach emphasizing personalized discussions between patient and provider that take into account a woman's unique health profile and individual needs.

Perimenopausal and postmenopausal women should have a conversation with their health care provider to determine if HRT is appropriate for them. Organizations like the North American Menopause Society (NAMS www.menopause.org) foster the ongoing study of menopause and treatment options and help women find a doctor who focuses on managing menopause.

Andropause

Andropause refers to the natural age-related decline in testosterone levels in men. It's also known as male menopause, or "low T." The decline in testosterone levels gradually occurs over several years.

Andropause can cause fatigue, low libido, erectile dysfunction, and decreases in muscle mass, bone density, and cognitive function. Neurological symptoms of andropause include decreased memory, concentration, attention span, and planning, as well as depression and anxiety.

Testosterone replacement can help restore testosterone levels to normal and alleviate many symptoms of andropause. However, testosterone replacement therapy has risks, is not appropriate for everyone, and requires close monitoring. Determining if testosterone replacement is appropriate requires an in-depth discussion between the patient and their provider, taking into account the patient's medical history and individual needs, as well as the risks and benefits of hormone therapy.

Medications That Affect Memory

Statins

Statins treat high cholesterol and are the most commonly prescribed class of medications in the US. They play a role in promoting brain health by decreasing atherosclerosis. However, they can have side effects that negatively affect brain health. If you take a medication to control high cholesterol and its generic name ends in -*statin*, review the information sheet that comes from the pharmacy with your medication. You may notice "decreased CoQ10 levels" listed as a side effect.

At the beginning of the book, we discussed the brain energy crisis of Alzheimer's disease. Mitochondria are the miniature power plants inside cells that convert oxygen and sugar into energy. CoQ10 is a cofactor in this process, meaning it's a molecule that's needed to assist in the chemical reaction. Statins can contribute to the crisis by starving your mitochondrial power plants of CoQ10. If you take a statin, talk to your doctor about starting a CoQ10 supplement, if you aren't already taking one, to mitigate this potential medication side effect.

Medications That Affect Acetylcholine (ACh) Levels

Neurotransmitter imbalance is one of the core processes of Alzheimer's disease. Acetylcholine, or ACh, is an important neurotransmitter that brain cells use to communicate. It is important for memory and is low in the brains of people with Alzheimer's disease. The first medications developed to alleviate the symptoms of Alzheimer's—donepezil (Aricept), tacrine (Cognex), rivastigmine (Exelon), and galantamine (Razadyne)—were all designed to increase ACh levels in the brain. Normal Ach levels are associated with normal cognitive function.

Medications that Lower ACh

On the opposite side of the spectrum are medications that lower ACh, either as their primary role or as a side effect. Medications that treat urinary incontinence, antihistamines, and some antidepressants can lower ACh levels in the brain and lead to memory impairment.

Medications for Urinary Incontinence

The brain and the bladder are at odds. To help memory, you want to increase ACh. However, if you want to settle down the bladder so you don't have accidents, you want to block ACh. This is a problem because the folks most likely to have challenges with urinary incontinence are in the age demographic at highest risk of developing dementia. The medications that treat bladder issues vary greatly as to how much they lower ACh in the brain. If you are taking a medication to treat bladder symptoms and you want to do everything you can to keep your brain functioning at its prime level, talk to your provider to make sure you are taking medicines that cause the least cognitive side effects possible.

Antihistamines

Antihistamines are great for getting allergies under control. Unfortunately, first-generation antihistamines—such as diphenhydramine, doxylamine, and chlorpheniramine—easily cross the BBB, where they can cause memory loss and confusion due to their ACh-lowering activity. Many first-generation antihistamine medications are available over the counter without a prescription, and that means your provider may not be aware that you're taking them. Keep your provider in the loop as to all supplements and nonprescription medications you take.

There are two reasons we become more sensitive to the ACh-lowering side effects of antihistamines as we age.

First, our natural ACh levels decrease mildly as we age, so it doesn't take as much to block ACh and cause symptoms. In addition, the body doesn't break down these medicines as quickly as it did earlier in life. That means the dose you tolerated well in the past now may stay in your system longer and make you spacey, distractable, or even goofy as you enter midlife and beyond.

If you take an over-the-counter antihistamine that contains diphenhydramine, doxylamine, or chlorpheniramine, your doctor or pharmacist may have a better option that is less likely to affect your ACh levels.

Second-generation antihistamines—such as loratadine (Claritin), cetirizine (Zyrtec), and fexofenadine (Allegra)—were developed to provide effective relief from allergies while minimizing undesirable side effects, like sedation and confusion. They don't cross the BBB, so they don't affect the ACh neurotransmitter system like the first-generation antihistamines do.

Antidepressants

The last group of medications that can lower ACh are older antidepressants, such as amitriptyline and imipramine. Fortunately, these medications are rarely used for depression these days. They have been replaced by newer antidepressants that are less likely to lower ACh levels. However, doctors still prescribe these medicines to treat other conditions, like migraines and nerve pain. Although the doses prescribed for those uses are usually much lower than the antidepressant doses, it is still important to discuss this topic with your provider if you are taking these medications, no matter the reason.

Traumatic Brain Injury

Over the past two decades, there has been a dramatic shift in the awareness of brain injury as a risk factor for Alzheimer's disease. Professional athletes suffering from chronic traumatic encephalopathy (CTE) have come into the spotlight after years of retirement. Repetitive concussions that were once ignored are now understood to increase the risk of dementia and severe psychiatric symptoms later in life.

I have evaluated dozens of former professional football players suffering from the remote brain consequences of trauma sustained decades earlier. Years ago, concussion was underrecognized. Players continued to participate while concussed and still seeing stars. I've met more than one player who was so confused, he tried to huddle with the opposing team and still was not removed from play.

Concussion guidelines are now in place for all levels of sports, from amateur through professional, kids through adults. It is critically important to follow these guidelines to minimize the possibility of reinjury.

Protective gear, including helmets, should be worn while participating in sports or while at work if there are potential hazards in your workplace.

Falls become a significant source of head trauma as we move into midlife and beyond. There are many things you can do to minimize the risk of falls. Exercising helps you maintain strength, balance, and coordination. Keep up to date with yearly checkups to identify any medical conditions that can increase the risk of falls. Assess your home, and remove any tripping hazards, like loose area rugs.

Take Action: Tasks, Goals, and Mini Habits

Address general medical concerns and optimize health

As you go through the list below, make a line through all the goals you've already accomplished or that don't apply to you.

Assess hydration and electrolyte status

- ☐ If you aren't drinking your daily goal for water that you set in Chapter 6, set a new list of mini habits to get back to your goal.
- ☐ If you participate in intense workouts, consider replacing electrolytes lost due to excessive sweat.

Consider vascular health

- ☐ Check your blood pressure. Use a free machine at your local pharmacy to see what your blood pressure runs when you are living your regular day-to-day life. You may find that it's different from what it runs when you are at your doctor's office. If the machine tells you it's abnormal, make an appointment to see your doctor ASAP.

☐ Revisit sugar intake. Are you still keeping it low? If not, refer to the tasks and habits at the end of Chapter 7, and get your intake back to the AHA goals.

Get up to date with medical visits

☐ If you're due for a checkup with your doctor, commit to calling this week to make an appointment.

☐ Make a list of things from this chapter you would like to address at that visit, including routine screening labs and any additional concerns based on conditions you or a first-degree relative has that were mentioned in the chapter. Discuss any medications you are taking and any concerns about potential cognitive side effects.

Have your hearing checked

☐ Schedule a hearing screening.

Practice good dental hygiene

☐ If you've fallen out of the habit of flossing your teeth, set up a streak to floss once daily.

☐ The next week, set up a streak to floss twice daily.

- [ ] If you're due for a visit with your dentist, call this week to schedule an appointment.

Talk to your provider about hormones

- [ ] Women: If you are perimenopausal or postmenopausal, talk to your doctor about menopause. If you don't have a provider who manages the symptoms of menopause, visit www.menopause.org.
- [ ] Men: If you are concerned about low testosterone, discuss it with your provider.

Review your medications

- [ ] Review the side effect profiles for your medications, both prescription and over the counter. Discuss any concerning side effects with your pharmacist or medical provider.
- [ ] Each time you add a new medication to your regimen, be sure to go over the side effects in the same way.
- [ ] If you are over 60, ask your provider to cross-reference your medications with the Beers Criteria at your next health checkup. This is a list that identifies medications associated with a higher risk of side effects in older individuals. This will help you and your doctor determine if your medications are still the most appropriate ones for you.

BRAIN HEALTH ACTION PLAN

- ☐ If you take any of the prescription or OTC medications listed in this chapter that can lower ACh, discuss your concerns with your medical provider.

- ☐ If you take a statin, ask your pharmacist to print out the information sheet for your particular medication. Review the sheet to see if low CoQ10 is a known side effect. If so, discuss CoQ10 supplementation with your provider.

Avoid brain injury

- ☐ If you participate in contact sports, wear protective equipment and follow concussion protocols.

- ☐ Wear helmets when recommended at work and while participating in sports like bicycling and skating.

- ☐ Continue the exercise habit you built in Chapter 12.

- ☐ Keep up with annual checkups with your medical provider to screen for conditions that can increase your risk of falls.

- ☐ Assess your home for tripping hazards. Consider adding nightlights if you get up in the middle of the night.

Notes

[1] Sheldon Weinbaum, Limary M. Cancel, Bingmei M. Fu, John M. Tarbell, "The Glycocalyx and Its Role in Vascular Physiology and Vascular Related Diseases," Cardiovasc Eng Technol 12, no. 1 (February 2021):37–71, https://doi.org/10.1007/s13239-020-00485-9.

[2] Nikita P. Patil, Almudena Gómez-Hernández, Fuming Zhang, Limary Cancel et al., "Rhamnan sulfate reduces atherosclerotic plaque formation and vascular inflammation," Biomaterials 291 (December 2022):121865, https://doi.org/10.1016/j.biomaterials.2022.121865.

[3] Nishikawa Masakatsu, Mitsui Masayuki, Umeda Koji, Kitaoka Yoshikuni, Takahashi Yoshie, Tanaka Shigeo, "Effect of sulfated polysaccharides extracted from sea alga (Monostroma latissium and Monostroma nitidum) on serum cholesterol in subjects with borderline or mild hypercholesterolemia," J New Rem Clin 55 (2006):1763–1770.

[4] Karen M. Rodrigue, "Contribution of cerebrovascular health to the diagnosis of Alzheimer disease," JAMA Neurol 70 (2013): 438–9, https://doi.org/10.1001%2Fjamaneurol.2013.1862.

[5] Livingston, Huntley, et al., "Dementia prevention, intervention, and care."

[6] Michael Roerecke, Janusz Kaczorowski, Sheldon W. Tobe, Gerrit Gmel, Omer S. M. Hasan, and Jürgen Rehm, "The effect of a reduction in alcohol consumption on blood pressure: a systematic review and meta-analysis," Lancet Public Health 2, no. 2 (February 2017):e108–e120, https://doi.org/10.1016/S2468-2667(17)30003-8.

[7] Yiqiu Zheng, Shengnuo Fan, Wang Liao, Wenli Fang, Songhua Xiao, and Jun Liu, "Hearing impairment and risk of Alzheimer's disease: a meta-analysis of prospective cohort studies," Neurol Sci 38, no. 2 (February 2017):233–239, https://doi.org/10.1007/s10072-016-2779-3.

[8] Brian Sheng Yep Yeo, et al., "Association of Hearing Aids and Cochlear Implants With Cognitive Decline and Dementia: A Systematic Review and Meta-analysis," JAMA Neurol 80, no. 2 (February 2023):134–141, https://doi.org/10.1001/jamaneurol.2022.4427.

[9] Muhammed Amer and Rehan Qayyum, "Relation between serum 25-hydroxyvitamin D and C-reactive protein in asymptomatic adults

(from the continuous National Health and Nutrition Examination Survey 2001 to 2006)," Am J Cardiol 109, no. 2 (January 2012):226–30, https://doi.org/10.1016/j.amjcard.2011.08.032.

[10] Marcus O. W. Grimm, Andrea Thiel, et al., "Vitamin D and Its Analogues Decrease Amyloid-β (Aβ) Formation and Increase Aβ-Degradation," Int J Mol Sci 18, no. 12 (December 2017):2764, https://doi.org/10.3390/ijms18122764; Ching-I Lin, Yi-Chen Chang, et al., "1,25(OH)2D3 Alleviates Aβ(25-35)-Induced Tau Hyperphosphorylation, Excessive Reactive Oxygen Species, and Apoptosis Through Interplay with Glial Cell Line-Derived Neurotrophic Factor Signaling in SH-SY5Y Cells," Int J Mol Sci 21, no. 12 (June 2020):4215, https://doi.org/10.3390/ijms21124215.

[11] Thomas J. Littlejohns, William E. Henley, et al., "Vitamin D and the risk of dementia and Alzheimer disease," Neurology 83, no. 10 (September 2014):920–8, https://doi.org/10.1212%2FWNL.0000000000000755.

[12] Maryam Ghahremani, Eric E. Smith, Hung-Yu Chen, Byron Creese, Zahra Goodarzi, and Zahinoor Ismail, "Vitamin D supplementation and incident dementia: Effects of sex, APOE, and baseline cognitive status," Alzheimer's Dement., no. 15 (2023):e12404, https://doi.org/10.1002/dad2.12404.

[13] Rebekah S. Vest and Christian J. Pike, "Gender, sex steroid hormones, and Alzheimer's disease," Horm Behav 63 (2013):301–307, https://doi.org/10.1016/j.yhbeh.2012.04.006.

[14] James H. Clark, "A critique of Women's Health Initiative Studies (2002–2006)," Nucl Recept Signal 30, no. 4 (October 2006):e023, https://doi.org/10.1621/nrs.04023.

[15] Jacques E. Rossouw, Garnet L. Anderson, et al., "Writing Group for the Women's Health Initiative Investigators. Risks and benefits of estrogen plus progestin in healthy postmenopausal women: principal results From the Women's Health Initiative randomized controlled trial," JAMA 288, no. 3 (July 2002):321–33, https://doi.org/10.1001/jama.288.3.321.

[16] Noor Ali, Rohab Sohail, Syeda Rabab Jaffer, et al., "The Role of Estrogen Therapy as a Protective Factor for Alzheimer's Disease and Dementia in Postmenopausal Women: A Comprehensive Review of the Literature," Cureus 15, no. 8 (August 2023):e43053, https://doi.org/10.7759%2Fcureus.43053.

CHAPTER 15

The Mind-Brain Connection: Stress, Spiritual Wellness, and Depression

Stress and Cortisol

We are a stressed-out society. While some stress is necessary for survival and optimal function, our modern lifestyles produce stress levels that are higher than ever before. Elevated stress harms the brain by accelerating aging, increasing inflammation, and promoting oxidative stress. Most of the negative health impacts of stress are mediated through the hormone cortisol, which was introduced in Chapter 11.

Although cortisol is often called the stress hormone, it's not all bad. Cortisol plays an important role in keeping people safe. When you face a threat, cortisol kicks in as part of your fight-or-flight response. It signals changes throughout your body that help you move quickly to avoid danger. It also causes your liver to dump sugar into your system to provide a quick burst of fuel. Furthermore, cortisol diverts blood flow away from the gut and increases heart rate and blood pressure, which makes oxygen and sugar more readily available to your muscles for action. This great system helped humans respond to big threats (like being eaten by beasts) and was critical for human survival.

Even though most of us no longer face the same serious survival threats our ancestors did, our modern lives are often characterized by frequent stress triggers and worries that lead to a nearly constant release of cortisol. Consistently high levels of cortisol cause sugar cravings, poor digestion, high blood pressure, high blood sugar, fatigue, and poor sleep.

You'll recall from Chapter 11 that cortisol is supposed to vary throughout the day. It is higher in the morning, when you need a burst of energy to wake up, and then gets lower in the evening, when your energy needs decrease. Getting a break from the stimulating effect of cortisol is critical for resting and falling asleep. When chronically high levels of cortisol replace your normal fluctuating levels of cortisol, your health suffers. Years of elevated cortisol contribute to diabetes, high blood pressure, obesity, heart disease, and insomnia. Managing stress and lessening cortisol are key components of keeping the brain and body healthy.

Spiritual Fitness

Spiritual fitness is a new concept in holistic wellness that encompasses religious and spiritual involvement. It is increasingly recognized for its role in Alzheimer's prevention.[1] Spiritual wellness practices, like prayer, mindfulness, meditation, and yoga, promote resilience and coping mechanisms that help lower cortisol levels. In addition, they regulate many of the core processes of Alzheimer's disease and are shown to have a beneficial effect on cognitive function.

Prayer and Religion

Practicing faith can lower cortisol levels. Studies show that prayer can decrease depression and anxiety, and those who regularly engage in prayer maintain lower cortisol levels in stressful situations. Religiosity is also associated with higher levels of neuron-supporting BDNF, even in the presence of depression.[2]

If you have a faith life, continuing to foster and grow your religious practice can promote brain health. Just as we worked to optimize exercise in Chapter 12, consider gradually expanding your religious activities by adding a daily devotional, book study, or group study.

Spirituality

Spirituality can mean many different things. People may consider themselves religious and spiritual or spiritual but not religious. In this book, spirituality refers to seeking a sacred or higher power that connects all beings to each other and the universe. If you have a spiritual practice, continue to expand your practice to maximize the calming effects and brain health benefits.

Mindfulness and Meditation

You can practice mindfulness and meditation in the context of religious worship or spirituality. Or you can practice them with a focus on connecting mind and body. If you don't already have a religious, spiritual, mindfulness, or meditation practice, Kirtan Kriya meditation might be a great practice to start for managing stress and promoting brain health. Even if you already practice one of the types of spiritual fitness discussed above, once you read about the scientifically studied benefits, you may want to incorporate it in your action plan as well.

Kirtan Kriya (KK) is a type of meditation and mantra practice that involves chanting repetitive sounds—"Saa, Taa, Naa, Maa"—while performing repetitive hand movements for twelve minutes. This brief meditation exercise has widespread and profound positive impacts on brain health. KK's meditation-based effects on the brain include decreasing inflammation, increasing blood flow to memory structures, and increasing brain volume.[3] People who consistently practice KK experience improved sleep, increased well-being, decreased anxiety, decreased depression, and improved memory.[4]

To get started, you can find an instructional video on YouTube or download the Kirtan Kriya instructions available from the Alzheimer's Research and Prevention Foundation.[5]

More Ways to Promote Well-Being, Manage Stress, and Reduce Cortisol

Seek Laughter

If none of the above suggestions feel right for you, how about laughing? Laughter decreases cortisol. Spend time with people who make you laugh, play silly games with family, and watch shows that make you laugh out loud.

Engage in Hobbies

Enjoyable activities that aren't tech centered can reduce stress. Crafting, knitting, writing, painting, working puzzles, and playing cards can lower your stress levels and also serve as brain exercise.

Write

Journaling can help you process emotions, gain insight, and solve problems. Externalizing your thoughts onto paper can interrupt negative cycles of rumination and help you develop a more balanced perspective. As a result, it reduces cortisol and depression. Incorporating a gratitude practice in your journaling, in which you acknowledge things you are grateful for, fosters a positive mindset and increases mood-boosting serotonin and dopamine in the brain. Shawn Achor brought attention to gratitude journaling in his 2011 TED Talk on happiness.[6] He highlighted a 2003 study that showed that listing three things you're grateful for at day's end can improve mood, outlook, and sleep.[7]

Limit Technology

Email and smartphones were designed to make our lives easier, but in many respects, they have done the opposite. Think critically about your relationship with your phone, take note of how often you check email, and ask yourself if that is necessary or excessive. Texts and emails can evoke twinges of stress, concern, and worry that bombard your system with cortisol all day long. Likewise, evaluate your use of social media and the emotions it triggers. Take a step back and set aside tech-free time in your day. Although people often use work breaks to scroll social media, consider setting aside your lunch hour as a tech-free time to enjoy lunch, talk with coworkers, and/or take a walk.

Eat Foods That Reduce Cortisol

Some foods can help decrease your cortisol levels. Try Brazil nuts, avocados, leafy greens, black and green teas, bananas, pears, and dark chocolate. Ideally, concentrate on using the first six items listed to crowd out less healthy choices, and reserve dark chocolate as a treat.

Deeper Dive into the Mind-Brain Connection: Depression

Depression in Early Adulthood and Midlife

Studies consistently show that depression in early adulthood or midlife doubles the risk of getting Alzheimer's disease and related dementias.[8] Early identification and treatment of depression is essential to reduce this risk. Depression shrinks the hippocampi, the primary short-term memory structures on each side of the brain, through several different mechanisms. Here's how that happens:

High cortisol: Chronic stress and depression both lead to chronic elevated cortisol levels. When scientists give animals high levels of cortisol, it damages their hippocampi. Memory cells in each hippocampus die off and are replaced by toxic amyloid plaques,[9] just like the ones Dr. Alzheimer saw in the very first Alzheimer's disease patient.

Low cerebral blood flow: Brain imaging studies show that in depression, there is decreased blood flow to the brain's hippocampi.[10] Reduced blood flow means reduced delivery of nutrients and less waste removal, which damages memory cells and causes shrinkage.

Inflammation: People suffering from depression have high levels of compounds called cytokines that increase brain inflammation and decrease new neuron growth in the hippocampus. Cytokines also wreak havoc in several important neurotransmitter systems, decreasing levels of serotonin, dopamine, and glutamate.[11]

Decreased brain-derived neurotrophic factor (BDNF) activity: BDNF supports growth and survival of neurons, including memory neurons in the hippocampus. Scientists report that people who suffer from depression have measurably lower levels of BDNF than people who don't suffer from depression.[12] Without adequate BDNF support, the memory neurons are more vulnerable to damage.

Late-Life Depression and Dementia

So far, we have focused on depression in early adulthood and midlife since those are target ages for dementia risk reduction. But what about depression in later life? Depression and dementia are closely intertwined in seniors. In fact, it's difficult to study them separately because they have common causes and contributing factors: lack of exercise, decreased blood flow to the hippocampus, and shrinkage of the hippocampus. Many doctors opine that late-life depression is not a risk factor for dementia but rather an early *symptom* of dementia. They are concerned that deterioration of the hippocampus first results in depression on its way to producing symptoms of dementia.

Although treatment of depression in seniors is important for well-being, it is not clear if treatment at this stage reduces risk of dementia as convincingly as treating it earlier in life does.

Another illustration of the close relationship between depression and dementia is a condition called **pseudodementia of depression**. In seniors, untreated moderate-to-severe depression can lead to profound cognitive impairment that mimics dementia. Distinguishing between the two is challenging for doctors because both conditions exhibit similar symptoms, such as memory loss and difficulty concentrating. Doctors rely on the patient's history and brain imaging, like MRIs, to differentiate between the two. The ultimate diagnosis often depends on whether or not cognitive symptoms improve with antidepressant treatment.

Despite similar outward symptoms, the underlying brain processes are different. At a cellular level, the neurons in Alzheimer's disease are damaged and dying, while pseudodementia features intact but dysfunctional neurons. Pseudodementia is considered a reversible cause of cognitive impairment, as antidepressant treatments can restore normal neuron function.

Take Action: Tasks, Goals, and Mini Habits

Cultivate well-being

- ☐ If you are spiritual or religious, brainstorm three ways you can increase your practice. Consider devoting more time, gaining deeper knowledge, or studying with a group.

BRAIN HEALTH ACTION PLAN

- ☐ Did you try meditating in Chapter 11? If not, try an online guided mindfulness meditation during your evening wind-down.
- ☐ Try box breathing or 4-7-8 breathing when you feel your stress levels rise.
- ☐ Try an introductory 20-minute yoga class online.
- ☐ Try Kirtan Kriya meditation. Set a streak goal to practice it 2 days per week for the next month. Each month, increase the frequency of KK by 1 day per week until you are doing KK most days.

Mitigate cortisol

- ☐ Find laughter daily. Seek time with someone who makes you laugh, exchange jokes with your spouse, read a funny book, or watch a show that makes you laugh out loud.
- ☐ Set aside time for hobbies weekly. If you don't have a big enough chunk of time available to get much done, miniaturize this goal by clearing space for your hobby one day, setting up the supplies another day, and working on the hobby another day.
- ☐ Write. Put pen to paper and write whatever comes to mind. Experiment with writing at the start of the day and at the end of the day to see which is more effective at alleviating worry and gaining perspective.

- ☐ Watch Shawn Anchor's 2011 TED Talk on happiness: https://www.ted.com/talks/shawn_achor_the_happy_secret_to_better_work

- ☐ Start a gratitude journal, either as part of your daily journaling or as a separate activity during your evening wind-down routine. Reflect on and write down three new things you are grateful for each day, and write down one positive thing that happened to you that day.

- ☐ Incorporate foods that lessen cortisol into your afternoon snack: Brazil nuts, avocado, bananas, pears, and decaffeinated black or green tea.

Limit tech-related stress

- ☐ Assess your relationship with your phone. Are you spending more time looking at its screen than you'd like to or than you think is healthy?

- ☐ Review the time tracker on your phone to see how much time you are spending on social media. Think about the feelings that social media provokes. Set a goal to cut down usage.

- ☐ Set aside an hour of tech-free time daily.

- ☐ Set a time when you will stop using your computer and phone at the end of the day.

- [ ] Set a time in the morning before which you won't check email or social media (preferably 30 to 60 minutes after waking up).

Assess your mental health

- [ ] Take an online depression self-assessment, such as the one offered by Kaiser Permanente: https://healthy.kaiserpermanente.org/health-wellness/depression-care/assessment
- [ ] If you feel depressed or concerns are raised on the self-assessment, contact your provider immediately for guidance.

NOTES

[1] Shera Hosseini, Ashok Chaurasia, and Mark Oremus, "The Effect of Religion and Spirituality on Cognitive Function: A Systematic Review," The Gerontologist 59, no. 2 (April 2019):e76–e85, https://doi.org/10.1093/geront/gnx024.

[2] Bruno Paz Mosqueiro, Marcelo P. Fleck, and Neua Sica da Rocha, "Increased Levels of Brain-Derived Neurotrophic Factor Are Associated With High Intrinsic Religiosity Among Depressed Inpatients," Front Psychiatry 10 (September 2019):671, https://doi.org/10.3389%2Ffpsyt.2019.00671.

[3] Kim E. Innes, Terry Kit Selfe, "Meditation as a therapeutic intervention for adults at risk for Alzheimer's disease - potential benefits and underlying mechanisms," Frontiers in psychiatry 5, no. 40 (April 2014) https://doi.org/10.3389/fpsyt.2014.00040.

[4] Dharma Singh Khalsa and Andrew B. Newberg, "Spiritual Fitness: A New Dimension in Alzheimer's Disease Prevention," J Alzheimers Dis 80, no. 2 (2021):505–519, https://doi.org/10.3233/jad-201433.

[5] Visit this link to access the instructions: https://alzheimersprevention.org/research/kirtan-kriya-yoga-exercise/

[6] TED, "The happy secret to better work | Shawn Achor," YouTube.com, February 1, 2012, https://www.youtube.com/watch?v=fLJsdqxnZb0.

[7] Robert A. Emmons and Michael E. McCullough, "Counting blessings versus burdens: an experimental investigation of gratitude and subjective well-being in daily life," Journal of personality and social psychology 84, no. 2 (2003):377–89, https://doi.org/10.1037//0022-3514.84.2.377.

[8] Amy L. Byers and Kristine Yaffe, "Depression and risk of developing dementia," Nature reviews Neurology 7, no. 6 (May 2011):323–31, https://doi.org/10.1038/nrneurol.2011.60; Holly Elser, Erzsébet Horváth-Puhó, et al., "Association of Early-, Middle-, and Late-Life Depression With Incident Dementia in a Danish Cohort," JAMA Neurol 80, no. 9 (2023):949–958, https://doi.org/10.1001/jamaneurol.2023.2309.

[9] Kim N Green, et al., "Glucocorticoids increase amyloid-beta and tau pathology in a mouse model of Alzheimer's disease," The Journal of neuroscience: the official journal of the Society for Neuroscience 26, no. 35 (2006):9047–56, https://doi.org/10.1523/JNEUROSCI.2797-06.2006.

[10] Joshua Chiappelli et al., "Depression, stress and regional cerebral blood flow," Journal of cerebral blood flow and metabolism: official journal of the International Society of Cerebral Blood Flow and Metabolism 43, no. 5 (2023):791–800, https://doi.org/10.1177/0271678X221148979.

[11] Andrew H Miller et al., "Cytokine targets in the brain: impact on neurotransmitters and neurocircuits," Depression and anxiety 30, no. 4 (2013):297–306, https://doi.org/10.1002/da.22084.

[12] Eero Castrén and Masami Kojima, "Brain-derived neurotrophic factor in mood disorders and antidepressant treatments," Neurobiology of disease 97, Pt B (2017):119–126, https://doi.org/10.1016/j.nbd.2016.07.010.

CHAPTER 16

Avoiding Toxins

Air Pollution

Air pollution is one of the twelve modifiable risk factors for dementia identified by the 2020 Lancet Commission. The term *air pollution* conjures images of smoggy, congested cities. As individuals, we don't have much ability to control outdoor air pollution.

Indoor air pollution also has an impact on brain health. Thankfully, as individuals, we have considerable control over our indoor environment. Practical strategies can help you mitigate exposure to indoor toxins at home and at work. Indoor air pollutants that we are concerned about in this chapter include particulates and volatile organic compounds.

Particulates include dust, pollen, pet dander, and tobacco smoke. These particles can trigger inflammation and oxidative stress in the brain. They also indirectly affect brain health by causing respiratory issues that lead to sleep disruption. Air purifiers that utilize high-efficiency particulate air (HEPA) filters effectively capture particulates and create healthier indoor environments.

Volatile organic compounds (VOCs) include chemicals like benzene, formaldehyde, toluene, and acetone that can evaporate into the air at room temperature. They come from a variety of household sources, such as paint, adhesives, cleaning products, furniture, air fresheners, and paraffin candles. VOCs are neurotoxins, and chronic exposure is implicated in the development of dementia.[1] To minimize exposure to VOCs, choose paints and cleaning products labeled "low-VOC" or "VOC-free." Use cleaning products in a well-ventilated space to help disperse any emitted VOCs quickly. Beeswax candles and coconut oil candles are lower-VOC alternatives to paraffin candles and air fresheners. You can also filter out VOCs from your home and office. HEPA filters do not absorb VOCs, but houseplants do! Plants play an important role in mitigating indoor air pollution through a process known as **phytoremediation**. Indoor plants that are recognized for their high rate of VOC filtration are spider plants, snake plants, peace lilies, and Boston ferns.

Alcohol

For years, I gave healthy brain talks in the community. People always perked up when they saw alcohol listed on my slide of things that were "good" for brain health. One of my favorite scientific studies to highlight was a 2013 study on champagne,[2] largely because I liked champagne. I also liked to think that any study endorsing my guilty pleasure had to be a great study.

In the study, researchers gave aged lab rats champagne for six weeks. They found that rats who had the human equivalent of one and a half glasses of champagne weekly did better than non drinking rats on memory tests. When they looked at the rats' brains, they found that their memory centers looked healthier. This was great news for elderly rats!

> "People love to hear good news about their bad habits."
>
> —John A. McDougall

The media made a huge leap in response to the study and claimed that drinking one to two glasses of champagne weekly helps prevent dementia, and that message went viral. This is not an accurate conclusion; instead, the study revealed that antioxidants found in champagne, called phenols and flavonoids, can have beneficial effects on rat brains.

Where all of this conclusion-drawing breaks down is that flavonoids and phenols are found in many places other than alcohol. Berries, citrus, tea, cabbage, onion, and kale contain flavonoids. Berries, olives, nuts, and coffee contain phenols. In my opinion, it would be interesting to see the results of another study in which researchers give one group of rats champagne and another group of rats an equivalent amount of phenols via nonalcoholic whole-food sources to see which group fares better. There is no indication that the brain needs exposure to the potentially harmful effects of the alcohol molecule in order to harness the beneficial effects of flavonoids and phenols.

Alcohol Is a Neurotoxin

Alcohol directly harms neurons, causing shrinkage in the hippocampus and the frontal lobes, which are involved in decision-making, personality, and inhibition.[3] Alcohol also promotes several of the core processes of Alzheimer's disease. It shifts neurotransmitter balance, enhancing GABA and inhibiting glutamate. The net result is slowed thinking, lack of coordination, and impaired decision-making. Alcohol also induces inflammation and oxidative stress in the brain.

It's hard to imagine how the small amount of beneficial compounds, like phenols and flavonoids, present in alcoholic beverages could outweigh the risks of exposure to alcohol itself. For example, researchers have also used animals to study a specific flavonoid called resveratrol, found in wine and fruit. At high doses, resveratrol decreases heart disease and brain disease in animals and increases their lifespan.[4] However, the amount of resveratrol it takes to achieve these positive health outcomes is the equivalent of drinking more than one hundred glasses of wine!

In a recent study in the *Journal of the American Medical Association*,[5] the amount of resveratrol that Europeans get from their diet and wine showed no benefit for heart health, brain health, or longevity. Using the positive compounds found in wine to justify drinking alcohol just doesn't hold up.

Moderation Was Key

We've known for decades that heavy drinking is bad for the brain. We thought moderation was the key to drinking alcohol without negatively impacting the brain. Some studies even suggested that moderate drinking—consuming two alcoholic beverages daily—is a healthier choice for the brain than not drinking at all. But a study of 25,000 people in the UK convincingly illustrates that as little as one drink daily (seven drinks per week) causes brain changes visible on MRI.[6] The type of alcohol doesn't seem to matter. Beer, wine, and spirits impact the brain similarly. Within the study, it remains clear that the damaging effects of alcohol increase as intake increases.

Crowding out and Interrupting

How much we drink matters. No matter where we start, decreasing alcohol intake proportionally reduces its damaging effects. Consider crowding out alcohol with nonalcoholic beverages. Start by crowding out one drink per week, then two per week, and keep going until you reach a level of drinking that is consistent with your overall health goals.

The interrupting strategy has long been part of social drinking and is called a spacer. This is a tried-and-true strategy to decrease alcohol intake. If you generally have several drinks when dining out or socializing, interrupt one drink per evening with a spacer of club soda or mineral water per evening. Depending on the length of the evening or event, you might consider having a spacer for every other drink.

It's difficult to talk about cutting back on alcohol. Family members, friends, and even doctors have difficulty approaching the subject. Drinking alcohol is relaxing, and everyone is dealing with stress. The recommendation to decrease drinking comes from a health perspective based on the most recent data, not a place of social or moral judgment.

Smoking

Thankfully, less than 12% of Americans smoke cigarettes today. Smoking increases the risk of stroke and Alzheimer's disease due to inflammation, oxidation, and decreased blood flow to the brain. The brain damage that smoking causes may be reversible, and the sooner you quit, the better chance you give your brain to heal from it. Smoking is one of the hardest habits to break. If you smoke and are considering quitting due to concerns about the impact on your brain and general health, reach out to your medical provider for guidance.

Vaping

So far, research on vaping suggests a higher risk of stroke in adults who use e-cigarettes than those who do not. Young adults who vape also have greater risk of anxiety and depression, both of which are associated with cognitive impairment.

Any type of smoking is a hard habit to break. Numerous books and programs deal with this subject, and I hope to stoke the fire of your motivation to quit. If you vape or smoke, the time to quit is now. Reach out to your provider for guidance.

Take Action: Tasks, Goals, and Mini Habits

Detoxify your home and office

- ☐ Look into HEPA filters that fit both your space and budget.
- ☐ When you shop for household cleaners, look for "low-VOC" or "VOC-free" options.
- ☐ Maximize ventilation by opening windows and utilizing fans or exhaust fans while using household products that contain VOCs to disperse them as quickly as possible.
- ☐ Avoid chemical air fresheners that contain VOCs.
- ☐ Opt for unscented beeswax candles or coconut wax candles instead of scented paraffin candles.

- [ ] Add houseplants to the places where you spend the most time, such as your desk at work and your bedroom. (If you are like me and don't have a green thumb, give yourself grace and replace them as needed!)

Minimize alcohol intake

- [ ] If you drink daily, crowd out 1 drink per day with mineral water with citrus, flavored mineral water, or even a low sugar kombucha. Every 2 weeks, crowd out another daily alcoholic drink until you reach your goal.
- [ ] When dining out and attending social events, use club soda or mineral water as a spacer to decrease overall alcohol intake.
- [ ] If you have been drinking alcohol during what is now your fasting period between dinner and bedtime, consider crowding it out with decaffeinated tea since that can also provide relaxation and ease stress. Plus, it doesn't have calories, so it won't delay the start of your fast.
- [ ] Consider going dry for a month and assess how you feel.

Quit smoking or vaping

- [ ] Spend some time reflecting on your habit. What are the benefits and costs of continuing to smoke or vape? What are the benefits and costs of quitting?

☐ Research local programs for quitting smoking or vaping.

☐ Make an appointment with your provider to discuss quitting smoking or vaping.

Notes

[1] Amjad Khan, Haafsa Kanwai, Salma Bibi, et al., "Volatile Organic Compounds and Neurological Disorders: From Exposure to Preventive Interventions," *Environmental Contaminants and Neurological Disorders* (2021):201–230, http://dx.doi.org/10.1007/978-3-030-66376-6_10.

[2] Giulia Corona, David Vauzour, Justine Hercelin, et al., "Phenolic acid intake, delivered via moderate champagne wine consumption, improves spatial working memory via the modulation of hippocampal and cortical protein expression/activation," Antioxid Redox Signal 19, no. 14 (November 2013):1676–89, https://doi.org/10.1089/ars.2012.5142.

[3] Anya Topiwala, Charlotte L. Allan, et al., "Moderate alcohol consumption as risk factor for adverse brain outcomes and cognitive decline: longitudinal cohort study," BMJ 357 (June 2017):j2353, https://doi.org/10.1136/bmj.j2353.

[4] In Soo Pyo, et al., "Mechanisms of Aging and the Preventive Effects of Resveratrol on Age-Related Diseases," Molecules (Basel, Switzerland) 25, no. 20 (October 2020):4649, https://doi.org/10.3390/molecules25204649.

[5] Richard D Semba et al., "Resveratrol levels and all-cause mortality in older community-dwelling adults," JAMA internal medicine 174, no. 7 (2014):1077–84, https://doi.org/10.1001/jamainternmed.2014.1582.

[6] Anya Topiwala, Klaus P. Ebmeier, Thomas Maullin-Sapey, Thomas E. Nichols, "Alcohol consumption and MRI markers of brain structure and function: Cohort study of 25,378 UK Biobank participants," Neuroimage Clin 35 (2022):103066, https://doi.org/10.1016/j.nicl.2022.103066.

CHAPTER 17

Recipes

Get a start on adding some new, healthy recipes to your weekly routine.

Breakfast

Overnight Oats

1 C milk of choice (dairy or nondairy)
1 C old-fashioned rolled oats

1. Stir together, cover tightly, and store in the refrigerator overnight.

Variations: Add flavor with ½ t vanilla extract, ¼ t cinnamon, or ½ t maple syrup; add creaminess by substituting ¼ C Greek yogurt in place of ¼ C milk; add protein, nutrients, and texture with 1 T chia seeds.

Baked Oats

2 C organic old-fashioned rolled oats
3 ripe bananas, mashed
2 apples, peeled and chopped
2 C milk (dairy or nondairy)
2 eggs, beaten
2 T melted butter
1 t baking powder
1 T pumpkin pie spice
1 t vanilla extract
½ C pecan pieces
½ C raisins

Non-seed-oil cooking spray or butter for baking dish

1. Preheat oven to 325°F. Lightly coat an 8" square glass baking dish with cooking oil spray or softened butter.
2. Mix the first 9 ingredients well. Stir in pecans and raisins.
3. Pour mixture into prepared baking dish.
4. Bake in the upper third of the oven for 45 minutes. Cool for 10 minutes before serving.

Natalie's Avocado Toast

Smash avocado on toasted and buttered sourdough bread. Sprinkle with pomegranate seeds. Drizzle lightly with honey.

Chia Pudding

¼ C chia seeds
1 C milk or milk alternative
Optional: ¼ t vanilla extract or cinnamon to taste

Mix ingredients and set aside. Stir again after 30 minutes and place overnight in the refrigerator.

Top with fresh or frozen fruit, toasted unsweetened coconut flakes, or low-sugar granola.

Baked Egg Pans

2 eggs
1 t heavy cream
¼ C toppings—any toppings you would use in an omelet, like cooked bacon, cubed ham, tomatoes, sautéed mushrooms, wilted spinach
1 t cheese—feta, Parmesan, mozzarella, or cheddar

1. Preheat oven to 400°F.
2. Coat inside of 6" ramekins, gratin dishes, or small ovenproof skillets with butter.
3. Add cream to each pan, then crack two eggs into each.
4. Add toppings and then cheese.
5. Place assembled baking dish onto a sheet pan and bake for 12 minutes or until egg whites are set.

Eggs in Edible Fruit Cups

2 eggs
2 tomatoes or bell peppers (yep they're fruits, not vegetables!)
½ t parmesan cheese
Pinch of herbs—basil, chives, or parsley
Optional: chopped cooked bacon, shredded cheese

Cut the top third off the tomatoes or bell peppers. Remove seeds and cores. Spray outside of your chosen fruits with avocado oil cooking spray. Crack an egg into each cup, top with bacon and shredded cheese as desired, and then with parmesan and herbs.

Baking methods:
Air Fryer: Preheat air fryer to 400°F. Spray air fryer plate with avocado oil. Place cups in the air fryer and air fry for 6–9 minutes, depending on how cooked you like your eggs. Cool for 5 minutes before serving.

Oven: Preheat to 350°F. Spray baking sheet with avocado oil, place cups on sheet, and bake for 25–35 minutes, depending on how cooked you like your eggs. Cool for 5 minutes before serving.

Leftover Frittata

A frittata is a great way to use up leftover meat, veggies, and whatever greens you have. It will provide breakfast for several days.

10 large eggs
1 ½ C shredded jack or cheddar cheese
½ C Parmesan cheese
¼ C meat of choice—suggestions include 5 slices of deli ham or turkey, cooked chicken (cubed or shredded)
2 T butter
2 T olive oil
½ t white pepper
4 green onions, sliced into rounds.
10 oz. greens—arugula, spinach, chard, or kale

1. Preheat oven to 350°F.
2. In a bowl, whisk together eggs and white pepper. Stir in cheese and meat.
3. Melt 1 T butter in an ovenproof skillet over medium heat; add 1 T olive oil. Add onion and cook for 2 minutes, stirring frequently. Add greens and cook until wilted.
4. Transfer greens to a colander and press out water. Stir wilted greens into eggs.
5. Add remaining butter and olive oil to the skillet and melt over medium heat to coat the pan. Pour in egg mixture.
6. Bake in oven for 20 minutes or until slightly puffy and set.
7. Remove from oven and let cool for 10 minutes before serving.

Lunch and Dinner

All recipes are 4 servings.

Weeknight Mexican Chicken Soup

2 T olive oil
1 lb. boneless chicken thighs, cubed
1 T taco seasoning
1 C frozen corn
1 C salsa
1 C black beans, rinsed and drained
32 oz. reduced-sodium chicken broth
Sprigs of cilantro for garnish
Tortilla chips for topping (optional)

1. In a large saucepan, heat olive oil over medium-high heat. Add chicken and cook, stirring frequently, for 6–8 minutes or until no longer pink. Add taco seasoning and continue to stir.
2. Add remaining ingredients and bring to a boil. Reduce heat and continue to simmer uncovered for 10 minutes.
3. Skim fat. Top with fresh cilantro and tortilla chips if desired.

Southwest Meatloaf

1 ½ lb. ground beef
¾ C crushed corn tortilla chips
1 large egg
15 oz. canned corn, drained
11 oz. chunky salsa
½ t salt
¼ t pepper

1. Preheat oven to 375°F.
2. In a large bowl, mix ground beef, tortilla chips, egg, corn, salt, pepper, and 1 C of salsa. Do not overmix.
3. Transfer mixture to a roasting pan; shape into a 10" x 5" loaf. Top with remaining ¼ C salsa.
4. Bake for 1 hour or until internal temperature reaches 160°F.

Thai Coconut Soup

1 lb. boneless chicken breast or thighs, cut into 1" cubes
14 oz. coconut milk (unsweetened)
14 oz. reduced-sodium chicken broth
Ginger
1 stalk of lemongrass, cut into 1" pieces
1 T freshly squeezed lime juice
1 C sliced mushrooms
1 T Vietnamese fish sauce
1 t Thai chili paste
Fresh basil leaves
Fresh cilantro

1. In a medium saucepan, combine coconut milk, chicken broth, lemongrass, and 6 quarter-size slices of fresh ginger. Bring to a boil.
2. Add chicken, mushrooms, lime juice, fish sauce, and chili paste. Reduce heat and simmer until chicken is opaque, about 10 minutes.
3. Discard lemongrass.
4. Garnish each serving with basil and cilantro leaves.

Seasoned Chicken Thighs

This is my favorite weeknight go-to recipe. I make a quadruple batch of the seasoning so I have it on hand in the pantry. When I've forgotten to plan dinner, I can still cook a tasty and healthy meal by just picking up a package of chicken on my way home from work.

Seasoning:
2 t onion powder
½ t dried thyme or oregano
1 t garlic powder
1 t smoked paprika
½ t white pepper
½ t cayenne pepper
½ t bouillon powder or salt

1. Combine all spices and store in an airtight container.

Chicken:
2 ½ – 3 lb. bone-in, skin-on chicken thighs
2 t salt

1. Preheat oven to 475°F.
2. Wash chicken thighs and pat dry with a paper towel. Salt chicken.
3. Sprinkle both sides with a generous amount of the seasoning mix.
4. Place thighs on a sheet pan and air-dry before baking. Alternatively, you can season the thighs the night or morning prior to baking and let them sit in the refrigerator uncovered until ready to bake.

5. Bake at 475°F for 20 minutes, then decrease temperature to 400°F for another 30 minutes or until the juices run clear and the temperature measured near the bone is 165°F.

Dutch Oven Lemon Chicken Tenders with Cauliflower

2 T avocado oil
2 lb. frozen chicken breast tenderloins
1 yellow onion, chopped
½ cauliflower
5 cloves garlic, chopped
1 t fresh thyme, chopped
¼ C lemon juice
3/4 C reduced-sodium chicken broth
1 t lemon rind, finely shredded
2 C fresh packaged spinach
¼ C sliced green onion

1. Preheat oven to 375°F. In a Dutch oven, heat avocado oil over medium-high heat. Add frozen chicken tenders and cook until golden brown, about 3–4 minutes per side. Transfer to a plate.
2. Add onion and cauliflower to Dutch oven, and cook until lightly browned—about 2 minutes. Add garlic, thyme, and ¼ t each of salt and pepper. Cook for another 30 seconds. Add lemon juice and stir, scraping pan drippings.

3. Return chicken to Dutch oven. Add chicken broth and lemon rind. Bring to a boil, then cover and transfer to oven.
4. Bake for 10 minutes or until chicken is cooked through (170°F). Remove from the oven, add spinach and green onion, replace the cover, and let stand for 2 minutes.
5. Serve with rice (optional).

Sheet Pan Gnocchi

1 lb. potato gnocchi (fresh, shelf-stable, or frozen)
2 pt. cherry tomatoes
12 oz. fresh ciliegine mozzarella balls (cherry-size), drained
12 oz. Italian sausages, cut into ½" slices
2 T avocado oil
½ t kosher salt
¼ t pepper
Fresh basil leaves

1. Heat oven to 400°F. Place cherry tomatoes and gnocchi on a rimmed baking sheet. Drizzle with avocado oil, then season with salt and pepper. Toss to combine.
2. Add sausage slices to the pan. Spread tomatoes, gnocchi, and sausage into an even layer.
3. Roast, stirring halfway through, until gnocchi are plump and some of the tomatoes have burst and caramelized, about 10 minutes. Remove from the

oven and add mozzarella balls. Toss to combine, again spread to an even layer, and roast for 3 more minutes.
4. Garnish with fresh basil leaves.

Thai Shrimp and Rice

1 lb. shrimp, peeled and deveined
1 ½ C black rice
1 C coconut milk (unsweetened)
1 ½ C water
¾ t salt
2 T olive oil
1 lime, cut into quarters
2 green onions, chopped
2 t fresh ginger, grated
5 stalks asparagus, cut into 1" pieces
1 T serrano pepper, finely chopped (optional)

Rice:
1. Combine rice, coconut milk, water, and salt in a medium saucepan. Bring to a boil.
2. Stir, reduce heat, cover, and simmer for 20 minutes or until tender.
3. Remove from heat and let stand covered for 10 minutes.

Shrimp:
1. Heat 1 T olive oil in a large skillet over medium heat. Add serrano and ginger. Cook for 30 seconds.

2. Add asparagus and increase heat to medium high. Cook for 4 minutes, then transfer to a plate.
3. Add 1 T olive oil to the skillet. Add shrimp in a single layer and cook, turning once, for 3–4 minutes until opaque.
4. Fluff rice, then add asparagus before serving. Top with shrimp and green onions, drizzle with lime juice.

Slow Cooker Balsamic Beef

1 ½–2 lb. chuck roast, boneless
1 C beef broth
½ C balsamic vinegar
1 T Worcestershire sauce
1 T soy sauce
3 T honey
3 t minced garlic

1. Season all sides of the roast generously with salt and pepper.
2. Place roast in slow cooker. (If time allows, brown all sides in a skillet with olive oil prior to placing in slow cooker.)
3. Combine all other ingredients in a small bowl and pour over beef.
4. Cook on low for 6–8 hours.
5. Remove beef from slow cooker. Use two forks to shred the meat or slice the roast against the grain. Return meat to the slow cooker and toss with sauce.
6. Serve with vegetables or potatoes, or on sandwich rolls.

Cabbage Pizzas

¼ C avocado oil
¼ C grated parmesan cheese
½ t onion powder
½ t garlic powder
½ t Italian herb mix
1 green cabbage
Cheese and toppings of choice
Salt and pepper

1. Heat oven to 425°F.
2. Cut four ½ inch thick slices from the center of the cabbage (imagine it's around the "equator" of the cabbage"). Set on a parchment-lined cookie sheet.
3. Combine the first four ingredients, brush mixture on both sides of the cabbage slices. Sprinkle with salt and pepper.
4. Bake for 30 minutes, or until golden brown.
5. Remove cabbage slices from the oven and top with sauce, cheese, and toppings of choice.
   a. Suggestions include: marinara sauce, mozzarella, and pepperoni; pesto sauce, mozzarella, and shredded chicken; feta, olives, and tomatoes.
6. Return cabbage slices to the oven and bake until cheese is melted and toppings are heated through.

Swordfish Kebabs

2 lb. swordfish, skin removed, cut into 1" pieces
1 pineapple, cut into 1" pieces
1 red onion, cut into 1" pieces
4 cloves garlic, finely chopped
1 ½ pieces of ginger, peeled and finely chopped
3 T avocado oil, plus more for grill grates
1 lime, juiced
½ t crushed red pepper
1 t pepper
1 t salt

1. In a medium bowl, combine garlic, ginger, lime juice, avocado oil, salt, pepper, and crushed red pepper.
2. Add swordfish to bowl and toss to coat. Cover and marinate in the refrigerator for 1 hour.
3. Heat grill to high.
4. Thread swordfish, pineapple, and onions onto skewers.
5. Cook skewers for 3–4 minutes or until fish is cooked through, turning occasionally.

Chai Tea Concentrate

30 black peppercorns
20 cardamom pods
10 cloves
½ t fennel seeds, chopped
4 black tea bags
½ t vanilla extract
3 C water
Dairy or nondairy milk

1. Crush peppercorns, cardamom, and cloves with a mortar and pestle.
2. Place crushed spices in a large saucepan, then toast over medium heat for 3–4 minutes. Add 3 C water and ginger. Bring to a boil, then remove from heat.
3. Add tea bags and steep for 5 minutes.
4. Remove tea bags.
5. Stir in vanilla and let stand for 1 hour.
6. Strain and discard solids. Store liquid in the refrigerator for up to 2 weeks.

To serve, mix 1 part chai concentrate to 1 part dairy or nondairy milk. Add minimal coconut sugar, maple syrup, or honey to taste.

APPENDIX A

Protein

Approximate protein content of some common foods. Values vary between brands, so check the nutrition label when possible.

Food	Protein Content	Serving Size
Almonds	6 g	1 oz.
Bacon	3 g	1 slice
Beef steak	23 g	3 oz.
Peanut butter	7 g	2 T
Chia seeds	4 g	1 oz.
Chicken breasts	36 g	4 oz.
Chicken thighs	28 g	4 oz.
Cottage cheese	13 g	½ C
Edamame	17 g	1 C
Egg, extra-large	7 g	per egg
Salmon	21 g	3 oz.
Greek yogurt	24 g	1 C
Hummus	2 g	2 T

Food	Protein Content	Serving Size
Pork tenderloin	22 g	3 oz.
Kidney beans	7 g	½ C
Shrimp	19 g	3 oz.
Tofu	7 g	¼ C

APPENDIX B

Fiber

The Mayo Clinic recommended daily fiber intake:

Women 50 and under: 25 grams

Women over 50: 21 grams

Men 50 and under: 38 grams

Men over 50: 30 grams

Approximate fiber content of some common foods. It varies between brands, so always check the nutrition label.

Food	Fiber Content	Serving Size
Chia seeds	13.5 g	¼ C
Bran	10.5 g	1/8 C
Almonds	10 g	½ C
Prunes	6 g	½ C
Split peas	22 g	½ C

Food	Fiber Content	Serving Size
Brussels sprouts	3.5 g	½ C
Flax seeds	14 g	¼ C
Seaweed	5.5 g	½ C
Popcorn	7 g	½ C
Apples	7.5 g	½ C
Lima beans	12 g	1 C
Lentils	16 g	1 C
Black beans	17 g	1 C
Whole wheat pasta	6 g	1 C cooked
Raspberries	8 g	1 C
Chickpeas	11 g	1 C
Barley	6 g	1 C
Pears	6 g	per pear
Avocado	14 g	per avocado
Blackberries	8 g	1 C
Peanuts	6 g	½ C

Reminder: When increasing fiber, do not increase more than 5 g per day, and drink plenty of water. Rapidly increasing fiber can lead to gastrointestinal distress.

APPENDIX C

Streak Tracker

The streak tracker below provides a framework for you to customize your streak goals and track your progress.

☐	☐	☐	☐	☐	☐	☐
☐	☐	☐	☐	☐	☐	☐
☐	☐	☐	☐	☐	☐	☐
☐	☐	☐	☐	☐	☐	☐
☐	☐	☐	☐	☐	☐	☐
☐	☐	☐	☐	☐	☐	☐
☐	☐	☐	☐	☐	☐	☐
☐	☐	☐	☐	☐	☐	☐

When you set up a streak that is not every day, outline or circle the boxes of the days you intend to do that activity. Place an "X" when you accomplish the task. This is how it might look when you're three days into a streak goal of walking for 5 minutes every weekday for two weeks.

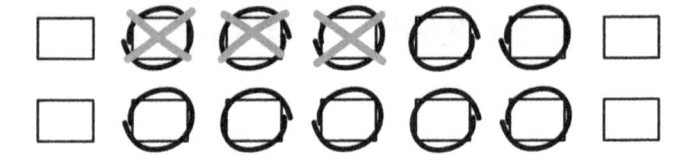

☐ ⊠ ⊠ ⊠ ◯ ◯ ☐
☐ ◯ ◯ ◯ ◯ ◯ ☐

ACKNOWLEDGEMENTS

Tremendous thanks to:

Graphic designer Jacqueline Pust for creating the interior artwork.

Catt Editing LLC for editing this manuscript.

Author Diane Stafford-Munoz who helped me understand what to write and how to write it.

Book coach Andrew Biernat, for setting the pace and getting me out of "Title Land."

Book Coach Allison Davis for picking up the baton and getting my manuscript across the finish line.

Our Bruin Woods family, the freshmamas, YC friends, and the Pacifica Christian and Liberty Baptist communities for your unwavering support and encouragement.

Colleagues Angela, Alicia, Jaime, Elena, Leslie, Nick, Jill, Mark, Jeff, Joe, and Richard: the many times you believed in me more than I believed in myself kept me going.

My inspired book study friends for your prayers and wisdom; and for helping me realize that writing non-fiction is a form of co-creating art.

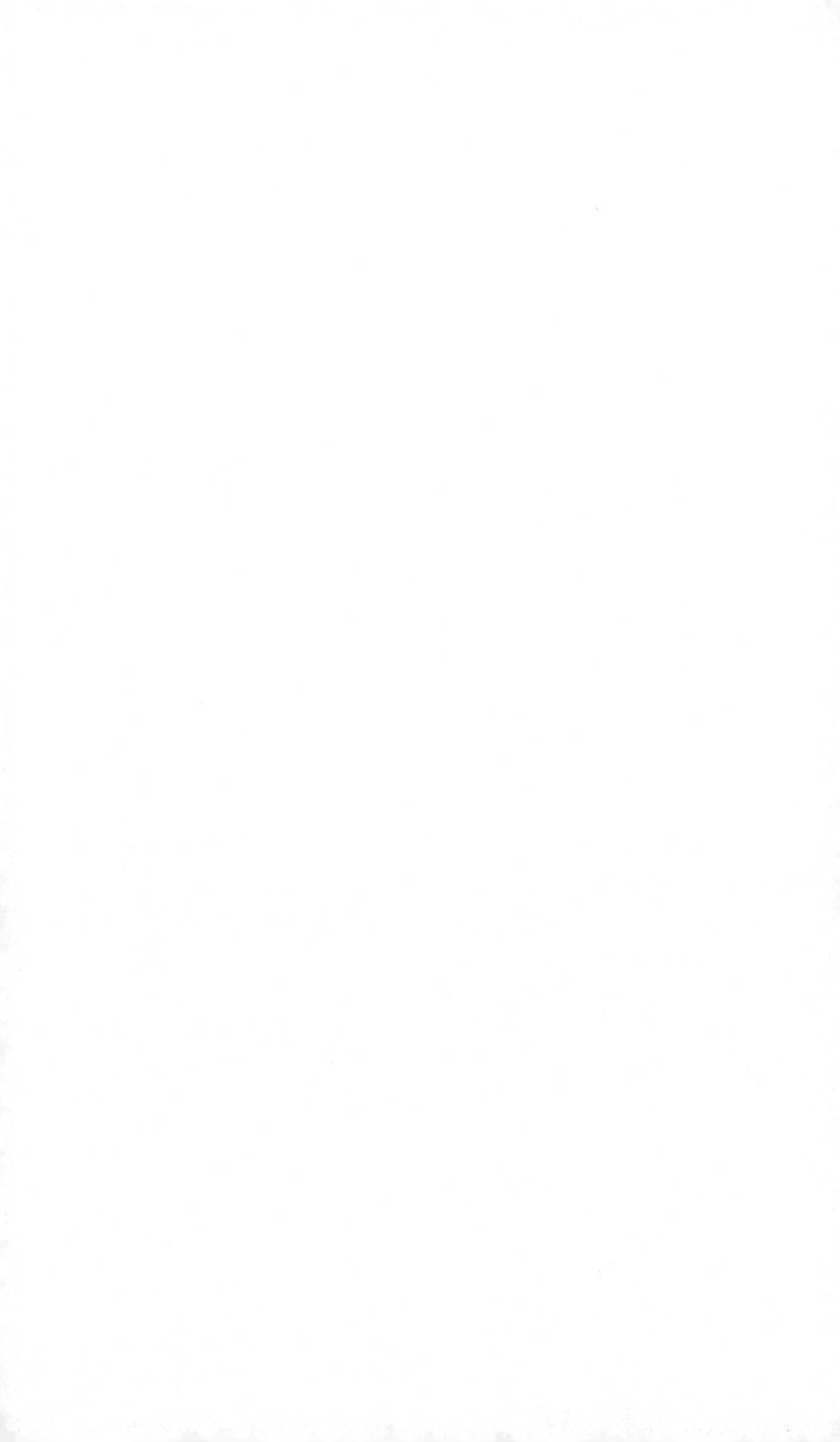

Made in the USA
Las Vegas, NV
21 June 2025